Dr. Payne's book is a valuable contribution to the current debate on the AIDS epidemic and its implications for American society and the church. It combines medical expertise and theological insight in a way that is all-too-frequently lacking in public discussions of this issue. I recommend it heartily to pastors, students, and people in our churches.

John Jefferson Davis, Ph.D., Professor of Systematic Theology and Christian Ethics, Gordon-Conwell Theological Seminary

I have followed the thinking, work, and writing of Dr. Payne and have always found him to be on the cutting edge in applying a Christian worldview to ethical issues in medicine. He is fresh and goes to the heart of the matter.

It is obviously more important to him to be Biblical than to be found acceptable to any group. He does not seek simply to reconcile two points of view, but seeks the balance of the Bible. Professionals and lay people alike will benefit from his work.

Joel Belz, Executive Editor, *World*, God's World Publications

Dr. Payne has revealed the Biblical framework as the only one in which the scientific data on AIDS can be properly understood. He reveals aspects of the epidemic that the news media has never considered and cannot comprehend.

We have the medical knowledge to deal with the epidemic, but we are not using it because we have ignored the Biblical principles that apply. Dr. Payne has shown us what those principles are.

Hilton P. Terrell, M.D., Ph.D., editor, *Journal of Biblical Ethics in Medicine*

If you want to know all about AIDS from one who understands both the medical and the Biblical data, this is the book for you. Every pastor, elder, deacon, and informed church member should buy it and keep it at hand. There is nothing comparable to it!

Jay E. Adams, Ph.D., Dean of the Christian Counseling and Educational Foundation

Other books by Franklin E. (Ed) Payne, Jr.:

Biblical/Medical Ethics:
The Christian and the Practice of Medicine

Making Biblical Decisions

What Every Christian Should Know About

The AIDS Epidemic

The Medical and Biblical Facts About AIDS

Franklin E. Payne, Jr., M.D.

Covenant Books

1991

What Every Christian Should Know About the AIDS Epidemic

Division of Covenant Enterprises
P.O. Box 14488
ugusta, GA 30919-0488.

ol H. Blair

ress Catalog Number: 91-72629
-3

States of America

Table of Contents

* The reader should see pages 36-38 to understand the relationship between HIV, AIDS-Related Complex, and AIDS.

To Jay E. Adams:

My beloved brother in Christ --
whose published and personal counsel has proved invaluable
in every area of my life.

With glory to God and deep gratitude to Jay.

Acknowledgments

No book is written without the enormous contribution of others. First, there are those teachers and authors who have molded and shaped my thoughts. Some have faded from memory, while others are vivid and compelling. God has been most gracious to provide me with some of His best for this purpose. Second, some people provide tangible and valuable contributions to make a specific work possible.

My greatest thanks go to my wife, Jeanne, who not only endures, but supports my uncommon ideas and projects.

Carol Blair has spent many diligent hours editing and improving everything in this book, as well as my two newsletters for the past three years. Her work has enhanced the quality of this book immeasurably.

Dr. Hilton Terrell, editor of the *Journal of Biblical Ethics in Medicine*, is always there to review everything that I write and to protest vigorously when I wander too far. Dr. Jim Fletcher has reviewed both my newsletters and other writings with faithfulness and skill. Dr. Peter Dailey has kept me accurate concerning virology, while Dr. John Jefferson Davis has provided theological oversight. Dr. Mike Felz provided review for early issues of my newsletters. Dr. Ronald Reed made a final medical review of this book.

Doctors Harold O. J. Brown, Jane Orient, and Herbert W. Titus allowed me to use their articles to improve this book substantially.

To all these I am deeply grateful for their time and expertise to make this book possible.

CHAPTER 1

AIDS: A Conflict Between Light and Darkness

AIDS (acquired immunodeficiency syndrome) is a unique disease. It is probably 100 percent fatal.[1] It is largely a disease of homosexuals, whose lifestyles are abhorrent to most Americans. It is a politically protected disease and one that has advanced the political agenda of the homosexuals. It is spread almost entirely by sexual immorality and drug abuse. And -- it is more, much more.

For Christians, AIDS is unique in another way: Its modes of transmission are strictly forbidden by God's Word. Yet, with more than 100,000 dead and 1 million infected with the AIDS virus, Christians are also called to show compassion to the suffering and dying. How then does one balance condemnation of sinful behaviors and at the same time be a Good Samaritan?

After a brief review of a Biblical perspective and a review of issues that will be discussed more fully in later chapters, we will see how the ACLU proposes the control of HIV (human immunodeficiency virus) in the hospital. By contrast, we will also see how one Christian physician took his stand "against the establishment" to protect himself and his co-workers.

Before reading further, however, it will be helpful for you to understand the relationship between HIV infection, AIDS-Related Complex (ARC), and AIDS (pages 36-38).

The Christian's Perspective

Christians must respond only within a knowledgeable worldview. We are engaged in a battle of light against darkness, but too often we only reflect secular attitudes and activities. Our worldview is Biblical and it is distinctive. God has told us that His Word sufficiently speaks to every issue.

> "All Scripture is given by inspiration of God, and is profitable for doctrine [teaching], for reproof, for correction, for instruction in righteousness, that the man of God may be complete, thoroughly equipped for every good work" (II Timothy 3:16-17, NKJV). See also II Peter 1:3.

Thus, our first response must be to see what the Bible says about the AIDS epidemic.

Now, those who have tried to handle ethical problems in this manner have found that the Bible is often silent on many subjects in its explicit statements. For example, the word *abortion* does not appear in the Bible,[2] but the subject of abortion is addressed by the Sixth Commandment (Exodus 20:13) and many verses that emphasize that life begins at conception (for example, Genesis 4:1; Ruth 4:13; and Psalm 51:5) and God's treatment of the unborn as individual persons (for example, Psalm 139:13-18; Jeremiah 1:5; and Luke 1:15).

The Westminster Confession of Faith describes the step whereby we can move from areas where the Bible is not explicit to identify the applicable Biblical principle. It tells us that a principle "by good and necessary consequence may be deduced from Scripture."[3] Deduction is the logical process that moves from statements (premises) to conclusions. If one's logic is proper, then such conclusions are as truthful as the statements themselves.

The formal process of logic is not usually stated in one's arguments and conclusions. Generally, it will not be stated in mine either. We should, however, be aware of the necessity of our reasoning from Scripture by this formal method to be certain of our position. The point here is that we must search for the Biblical principles that apply to the AIDS epidemic.

Sound Knowledge

The writer of the book of Hebrews exhorts Christians to

"have their senses exercised to discern both good and evil" (Hebrews 5:14b). This exercise calls for the Biblical application just described and an accurate understanding of the medical facts concerning HIV and AIDS. These medical facts are well-known, much more so than early in the epidemic when the cause of AIDS was unknown. The argument could be made that more research has been carried out on AIDS than any other infectious disease in the history of medicine.

Thus, the facts that are needed to make important personal and public decisions concerning this epidemic are known. "Sound knowledge" is the most critical response to be made, because it will determine the action that follows.

Compassion and Charity

The parable of the Good Samaritan (Luke 10:25-37), the picture of judgment based upon compassionate acts (Matthew 25:31-46), and many other verses make a solid case for the compassion of the Christian toward the poor, unfortunate, and downtrodden. Certainly, this response is needed towards those who are HIV-positive and AIDS patients. It includes *both* an offer of the Gospel and physical care (James 2:15-17). Yet, this response is only one part of the comprehensive response that is needed. Further, we should not neglect the care of those with "ordinary" diseases.

Homosexuality

The subject of AIDS is different from the abortion issue in that the Bible speaks explicitly about homosexuality, the subject that may be the most major issue for Christians concerning AIDS. It is a subject that is somewhat neglected by Christian writers and ethicists.

On the one hand, the Bible is clear that homosexuality is an abomination to God (Leviticus 18:22-30). It is contrary to the "one flesh" design for male and female in the beginning (Genesis 2:23-24). It is the bottom rung of the ladder of rebellion against God. That is, it is the point at which God "gives them (the rebellious ones) up" to the full extent of their wickedness (Romans 1:18-32). It is incompatible with heaven (I Corinthians 6:9-10; Revelation 21:8).

On the other hand, the Bible is clear that homosexuality is a forgivable sin. "And such *were* some of you. But you *were washed*, but you *were sanctified*, but you *were justified* in the name of the Lord Jesus and by the Spirit of our God" (I Corinthians 6:11, emphasis added). This verse clearly says that some had been saved out of their previous wickedness, clearly described in verses 9-10. Some of these were homosexuals. Also, there are former homosexuals today who give clear testimonies of their position in Christ *and their repentance from homosexuality*. The latter is as important as the former, because a continuing homosexual lifestyle for a professing Christian is incompatible with its Biblical condemnation.

The medical conditions associated with homosexuals are consistent with the Biblical picture of abomination. Homosexuals have a far higher incidence of sexually transmitted diseases than heterosexuals. They have what was once called the "gay bowel syndrome,"[4] which is a group of intestinal infections that are rare in the United States, but more common among homosexuals. In fact, the diagnosis of these infections in a male automatically causes a physician to consider that this patient is a practicing homosexual. Other infections that are more common among homosexuals than in the general population are hepatitis B, cytomegalovirus, and Epstein-Barr virus.

As a general rule, the presence of diseases associated with a lifestyle reflects its sin orientation. For example, alcoholism causes cirrhosis of the liver (the liver "dies"), degeneration of the brain, pneumonia, accidents, and gastritis (inflammation of the stomach). The associations of disease with homosexuality are considerable. (For more on homosexuality, see Chapter 5.)

Public Health

The Old Testament laws concerning regulation of certain diseases and quarantine seem to give the government certain authority over these areas (Leviticus 13-15). Thus, the responsibility does fall to the government to apply those public health measures that are necessary to limit the spread of HIV. This regulation of public health is not, however, without certain limits. For example, the widespread availability of abortion is now considered necessary for the public's health. Pro-life Christians, however, *strongly* differ with this position. Thus, even as we recognize the right and the responsibility of the government in this epidemic, we must realize its limitations.

This brief overview provides our introduction to this epidemic from a Biblical perspective. The task remains in the following chapters to discuss these issues more in depth. Before moving on, however, the following accounts contrast non-Biblical and Biblical approaches to AIDS. (For more on public health issues, see Chapter 11.)

The ACLU on AIDS

Harold O. J. Brown, Ph.D.[5]

In addition to taking a very active interest in "reproductive freedom," the ever-vigilant American Civil Liberties Union, through its AIDS (acquired immunodeficiency syndrome) and Civil Liberties Project, offers advice to nurses and other health-care workers. A growing number of physicians, operating room nurses, and other health-care workers have been demanding to be informed whenever they are dealing with an AIDS patient or non-symptomatic HIV (human immunodeficiency virus or "AIDS virus") carrier. Although AIDS is not highly contagious, ... once contracted, there is no treatment for it, and it is virtually certain to be fatal.

In consequence, surgeons and other operating room personnel are legitimately apprehensive when dealing with AIDS patients. Surgery always involves blood, as much emergency room treatment also does, and where sharp instruments, broken bones, and other items capable of causing cuts or puncture wounds must be handled under conditions of stress, surgical rubber gloves offer only partial protection. Nurses and laboratory personnel often draw and handle blood. It is not likely that a nurse will stick herself with the same needle that she has just used to draw blood, but if it happens and the blood contains HIV, she is in for some very serious trouble indeed. It goes without saying that if a nurse is aware that a patient is carrying HIV, she will exercise greater caution than the pressure of time and workload permit her to use with all her patients.

Timothy Bishop, staff counsel with the AIDS and Civil Liberties Project of the Roger Baldwin Foundation of the ACLU, offers the medical and nursing professions the advice that they should assume that *all* patients are infectious for HIV and other blood-borne diseases, such as hepatitis. Therefore, "they should use standard precautions such as gloves and masks with every patient." Most nurses work an eight-hour shift. Perhaps Mr. Bishop should try wearing a surgical mask and gloves for eight consecutive hours, just to get a little idea of what he is asking them to do. A contrary vote was offered by hematology professor Everett Bruckner, M.D., of Loma Linda, California, who stated that he always tries to avoid gloves and a mask at bedside visits, even with AIDS patients, except when performing a risky procedure, "for the sake of human warmth."

Bishop argues, "Studies suggest that it is counterproductive to identify patients known to be HIV-positive, because health-care workers may neglect to use standard precautions with other patients. That is very dangerous, because HIV tests produce 'false negative' results with some patients and others with the disease may not have been tested." There are about 50,000 active AIDS patients in the United States at this time, most of whom will be recognized as such when admitted to the hospital. If we take the generous estimate that there are 1.5 million HIV carriers in the United States today, this means that 0.6 percent of the population may carry HIV.

AIDS testing is supposed to yield a very tiny percentage of false positives; even if we assume 1.0 percent, then the chance that a hospital patient will be HIV positive but falsely identified as negative is 0.006 percent, or about one in 16,700. Admittedly these are crude estimates, but it is evident that the risks Mr. Bishop evokes are very small indeed. He would require nurses to approach several thousand non-contagious patients wearing gloves and masks for every single patient who might be contagious--thousands of unnecessary precautions for every instance when precautions would be called for--but in those cases the general precautions he advocates would not necessarily be adequate. *Cui bono?* Certainly the manufacturers of surgical gloves would benefit. But would the patients and health-care workers?

Confronted with a dental hygienist in mask and gloves, this editor asked her what precautions she would take if she knew that she were dealing with an AIDS patient (she has worked with a few). She answered, "The same as with everyone else, except that I would put on two pairs of gloves."

Because AIDS was closely identified from the first with homosexual conduct, which the major religions and much of the general public have long regarded as a perversion, apprehensions about AIDS, even in the form of normal medical and public health precautions, is taken as hostility to homosexuality, as "homophobia," and perhaps even as an "establishment of religion"-- one of the most dreadful things ever contemplated by the ACLU. No doubt such sentiments--prejudices, if you will--do play a role, but the fact remains that apprehension about AIDS is fully understandable as fear of a fatal disease and does not need to be interpreted in terms of "homophobia."

Perhaps it is fair to suggest that inasmuch as the ACLU is so vigilant and so ready to take extensive precautions lest any suspicion of an "establishment of religion" infect American life, it should be less judgmental when others want to take precautions concerning AIDS. After all, however bad an establishment of religion may be, it is not 100 percent fatal. AIDS is.

One Physician's Stand Against the Establishment

While the care of patients has many rewards, it also has its hazards for health-care workers. Perhaps, the greatest hazard is the workers' exposure to infectious diseases. A common means of exposure is the accidental puncture of the skin by a needle -- or "needle-stick." This type of accident may occur during the process of drawing blood, giving injections, or working with IVs (intravenous needles and other equipment). The greater the hurry or the inexperience of the person, the greater the chance of this injury. There is also significant hazard for those who "clean up," because needles, broken glass, and other sharp objects may be hidden in linen and other material.

It is common practice in many hospitals to have "on-the-job" injuries, including needle-sticks, evaluated and treated by the physicians who work in that hospital's own emergency room. Dr. Ronald W. Reed is a specialist in Internal Medicine who is one of those ER physicians at Reading Hospital in Reading, Pennsylvania.[6]

His hospital employs 3,000 people, and several are seen by the ER physicians each day for needle-sticks or other injuries from sharp objects that may have been contaminated with a patient's "body fluids." Since these injuries occur commonly and have many personal, social, and legal ramifications, a protocol is followed that includes checking the incident patient's blood for certain diseases, such as hepatitis B and syphilis, that might infect the exposed health-care worker.

After testing for HIV (human immunodeficiency virus) became available in 1984, Dr. Reed began to order it on these incident patients, as well. Logically, a health-care worker would want to know if he or she had been exposed to a potentially fatal disease, such as the virus that causes AIDS. He began to notice, however, that HIV testing of the incident patient was not listed on the protocol. He assumed that the omission was an oversight, since the test for HIV was still relatively new, and continued to order it.

In succession, however, he was soon visited by the Infectious Disease Control Nurse, the Chief of Infectious Diseases, the Hospital Staff President, and the President of the Hospital. The standard line was, "We have not worked out all the legal ramifications of HIV testing to make it part of the protocol." Then, he was visited by the hospital's attorneys. Finally, he was "clearly instructed not to order the tests."

However, *he could not and would not comply*, because it

violated standard principles of infection control that had been applied for decades and because such knowledge was crucial to the welfare of the injured employees. He was threatened with dismissal, but he continued his commitment to these principles. Several other ER physicians agreed with him and also continued to order tests for HIV in these situations.

Informed consent, *per se*, was never obtained. Upon admission to the hospital, however, each patient had signed a waiver that his blood could be tested if an employee was exposed to one of his "body fluids." No patient has brought legal action for this testing.

Later, hospital personnel presented a petition to the hospital authorities that such testing be made part of the protocol for needle-stick injuries. With this impetus, the protocol was changed to include testing of the incident patient for HIV. More recently, Dr. Reed learned that Reading Hospital is the only one in Pennsylvania where this protocol exists.

Thus, the matter stands at Reading Hospital. Its employees can be thankful that such a man as Dr. Reed stood his ground for their welfare and for standard principles for infectious diseases. A state law in Pennsylvania, however, is being considered that would require pre- and post-test counseling for anyone tested for HIV. These additional steps will likely cause some patients to refuse to be tested for HIV. Thus, if this bill is passed, Dr. Reed will have lost to the authority of the state, a common occurrence in the current milieu that protects the guilty and harms the innocent.

Notes and References

1. We still don't know whether AIDS will be 100 percent fatal because its long latent period and its recent onset in history have not allowed sufficient observation time for that conclusion. At this time, however, most evidence shows and most experts believe that its mortality will approach 100 percent.

2. Paul does refer to himself as "one born out of due time" (literally, an abortion), but not in the context of a moral application to a medical procedure (I Corinthians 15:8).

3. The Westminster Confession of Faith, Chapter I, 6. It is the basis of many conservative Reformed and Presbyterian churches.

4. "Gay bowel syndrome" is not a common term today in the medical

journals, probably because physicians are trying to be more "sensitive" about anything that might be considered to be derogatory towards homosexuals.

5. Dr. Brown is Professor of Systematic Theology at Trinity Evangelical Divinity School in Deerfield, Illinois, and co-founder and Chairman of the Christian Action Council. He has authored several books, including *Heresies*, *The Protest of a Troubled Protestant*, and *The Reconstruction of the Republic*. This article was taken from *The Religion and Society Report*, a monthly newsletter which he edits and which is published by the Rockford Foundation, 934 North Main Street, Rockford, IL 61103-7061. Reprinted by permission.

6. The following was excerpted from a talk that Dr. Reed gave at a medical ethics conference on April 28, 1990, in Philadelphia, sponsored by the Forum for Biblical Ethics in Medicine. It shows that *one* person can make a difference, not only in our fight to bring rational thinking to the AIDS epidemic, but in other areas where we should take a stand also. It is a "real life" account and not a theoretical "ought to." His entire talk is available on audio-cassette tape from Covenant Enterprises, publisher of this book.

CHAPTER 2

A Brief History of the AIDS Epidemic

A history of the HIV (human immunodeficiency virus) and AIDS (acquired immunodeficiency syndrome) is important because these two entities have only recently arrived on the scene of human history. The disease was unknown in 1980, attracted attention only in 1982, and had its cause (HIV) identified only in 1984. A worldwide crisis unknown in the history of mankind is unfolding before our eyes.

The whole scenario seems a sort of fictional documentary except for the stark statistics of those who are HIV positive, who have AIDS, and who have died. Furthermore, it is well-known that established public health measures have not been applied to AIDS, resulting in some costly and tragic mistakes. These mistakes were made by people who are charged to "promote the general welfare."

The Beginning

The story begins with rare diseases that became common. In June 1981, the first report of what would later be called AIDS appeared. Twenty-six cases of Kaposi's sarcoma (KS) and 15 cases of *Pneumocystis carinii* pneumonia (PCP) were reported in young to middle-aged, homosexual men.[1] Kaposi's sarcoma had been a rare cancer, seen predominantly in elderly men, and producing bluish, brownish or violaceous skin lesions and a long clinical course. It was rarely fatal. In these younger patients, however, 20 percent had died within 2 years of their diagnosis.

Pneumocystis carinii is the name of a protozoan, common to the human environment, but rarely known to cause pneumonia except in patients whose immune system is compromised by medications or disease. Again, these serious cases of PCP in young men were a striking contrast to the usually harmless nature of *P. carinii*. Both groups of patients were also noted to have significant abnormalities of their immune systems (a marked decrease in T-cells).

The common findings noted in these patients were their active homosexual lifestyles, concurrent or previous cytomegalic virus (CMV) infections, and butyl nitrate or other inhalant drug abuse (to get a "high"). A list of possible causes included the CMV, inhalant drugs, prescription drugs, amebiasis, Epstein-Barr virus, and a genetic predisposition.

Dr. Daniel C. William, one of the physicians who early reported these patients with KS, suspected "immunological overload--that rapidly sequential or concurrent infections with many pathogens may be paralyzing their immune systems."[2] Although he did not mention the possibility of a virus, his interpretation of the host susceptibility is still likely the single most important factor to infection with AIDS. Immune suppression is common to promiscuous homosexuals who have repeated, multiple infections, whether they are infected with HIV or not. (For more on homosexuals, see Chapter 5.)

In November 1981, there were 153 cases of these diseases in homosexuals and one woman! The numbers were beginning to increase alarmingly and to spread beyond homosexuals.

"Only the Tip of the Iceberg"

Dr. William proved to be something of a prophet. In his conclusion, he stated that these diseases were "only the tip of the iceberg" relative to the immunological overload that he attributed to repeated multiple infections.[3] His predictions were all too accurate!

The recommendations that appeared in the same article from two organizations of *homosexual* physicians provide an interesting perspective. You should note that these recommendations were made *before* anyone had any idea of the epidemic that AIDS would become -- or its cause.

> "Always exchange your name and telephone number to facilitate contact in case signs or symptoms of an STD (sexually transmitted disease) are later discovered."
>
> "Rimming[4] except in an *exclusively* [their emphasis] monogamous relationship should be eliminated from the activities of everyone who is not interested in getting amebiasis, giardiasis, shigellosis, *Campylobacter* bowel infections, or hepatitis A or B."

These recommendations confirm that homosexuals' earlier positions on confidentiality and contact tracing have been changed by AIDS. Also, if homosexuals had followed their own physicians' advice, many thousands would not be dead or infected with HIV today.

A Few Months Later

By September 1982, the name *AIDS* been given to this strange new syndrome, and 579 cases had been reported. ("Syndrome" is applied to a common group of symptoms in patients, and thus is a description, not a diagnosis of cause.) High-risk groups for AIDS now included both homosexuals *and* IV-drug abusers.[5] The total number included 3 hemophiliacs, 36 Haitian immigrants, and (about) 30 women.

"The three cases of *P. carinii* among hemophiliacs are alarming to some since they suggest the possible transmission of an agent through blood products, although as yet there is no evidence for this."[6] Two of these patients had already died.

Investigators were still considering the same possibilities as noted earlier. "Several researchers have hypothesized that a new strain of virus may recently have evolved, but there is no evidence of this. In any case, *it seems unlikely that a virus alone is inducing AIDS*"[7] (my emphasis).

A Few More Months

In January 1983, the debate over screening blood donors

began when an *ad hoc* advisory committee was convened in Atlanta at the Centers for Disease Control (CDC). This group represented "every group with an interest in the burgeoning epidemic," including the various blood banking organizations, government agencies, and homosexual groups.[8] "The goal of the meeting was to forward some consensus recommendations" for the U.S. Department of Health and Human Services.[9] It was a tense meeting.

> "... The meeting was going badly.... The blood bankers were worried about money and the costs of drawing new donors ... (and) all the reporters that were covering the conference.... FDA (Food and Drug Administration) representatives were also wary of the CDC.... Gay organizations sided with the CDC on surrogate (indirect) tests of blood but opposed taking any action to screen blood donors, saying the screening would pose serious civil rights questions.... Hemophiliac organizations were stunned by the gay perspective. What about a hemophiliac's right to life? ... The (non-profit) blood bankers ... (became) resolutely opposed to blood testing, arguing almost solely on fiscal grounds.... With the fear of direct competition for their market, the spokesman for Alpha Therapeutic Corporation (a for-profit banker) announced that his firm ... would immediately begin screening donors and exclude all people in high-risk groups.... The meeting adjourned with no recommendation or agreed-upon course of action."[10]

These representatives had probably faced their finest hour *and failed*. It would be more than two years later before testing of the blood supply became mandatory. Various measures were voluntarily instituted by some blood banking groups, but rarely because of their concern for the protection of recipients. Noted reasons were the threat of competition from other blood banks who *did* institute screens and lawsuits by patients who might become infected via blood transfusions.[11]

By March 4, 1983, over <u>1200 cases</u> of AIDS had been

reported. Risk groups were expanded to include hemophiliacs, all sexual partners of patients with AIDS, sexual partners of individuals at increased risk for AIDS, and babies born to mothers with AIDS.

The AIDS Virus Is Discovered: By Whom?

On April 23, 1984, at a specially called news conference in Washington, D.C., the discovery of the etiologic agent for AIDS was announced.[12] At the time it was called HTLV-III (human T-cell lymphotrophic virus) because it was the third retrovirus (see below) to be discovered in humans. The immediate credit was given almost entirely to Dr. Robert C. Gallo of the National Cancer Institute (NCI).

In late 1985, however, the Pasteur Institute in France filed suit against the NCI.[13] The suit asked for a share of the royalties that the NCI was getting from its blood-test patent, but "the scientific community understood that the French were really suing for the full recognition that had been denied them" (that is, the discovery of the AIDS virus).[14]

The facts about this dispute may never be known. It seems, however, that Dr. Gallo did collaborate with Dr. Luc Montagnier of the Pasteur Institute on early research. As Dr. Gallo tells it, the French actually identified the virus but could not do the research to "prove" it to the scientific community.[15] Therefore, the French were initially given little or no credit, prompting their lawsuit.

The heads of both nations, Presidents Ronald Reagan and Jacques Chirac, eventually settled the controversy in a White House ceremony that made the researchers *co-discoverers* of the AIDS virus.[16] (That, my friends, is the highest level of arbitration!)

Retrovirology: A Fortuitous Science

DNA (the genetic blueprint for every cell in the human body) was mapped out only in 1953. Viruses were an essential part of DNA research from the beginning, because they are almost pure genetic material. Some viruses are RNA (the "second" kind of genetic material) and others, DNA. Most viruses reproduce by copying their own DNA.

Retroviruses are different, however, because they contain an enzyme (reverse transcriptase) that allows their conversion from RNA to DNA. Hence, they are called "retro" (reverse) viruses. Their DNA is then integrated into the DNA of their host cells. (Viruses live only within other living cells.) Linked with the DNA in this way, the exact viral particles can then be reproduced in mass quantities.

The study of retroviruses began in 1970. They were not thought to infect humans until Dr. Gallo discovered the first one, HTLV-I, in 1978. This field was so narrowly focused that it almost faltered in the mid-1970s. If AIDS had appeared a decade earlier, the causative agent might have remained a mystery for a long time.

Thus, in a sense, AIDS appeared almost coincidentally with the ability of science to discover its causative agent. Was this a "fluke" of history, or God's intention? What do you think?

Corruption - All?

While the homosexuals, and to a lesser extent the IV-drug abusers, comprise the greater portion of AIDS patients, scientists, government officials, and other administrators have complicated the epidemic by their own brand of moral corruption and selfishness. Should we expect anything else? Moral corruption, much as leaven does, spreads throughout the whole. We err if we consider that any part is any less affected. Any reformation must therefore affect the whole as well.

Bathhouses Close

On October 9, 1984, Dr. Merv Silverman, director of the Public Health Department of San Francisco, ordered that 14 bathhouses be closed.

> "The expected gay outcry that had so paralyzed the health department and intimidated politicians never

> happened.... Within a year of Silverman's order, baths were also closed in New York and Los Angeles.... Later, everybody agreed the baths should have been closed sooner."[17]

Three years earlier, public health officials *and* some homosexual leaders had warned of the dangers associated with such promiscuous sexual practices (above), but their warnings mostly went unheeded. At the end of 1984, 4686 cases of AIDS had been officially reported. Some 6.4 percent were women.

Heterosexual Transmission

A strange phenomenon was apparent in the worldwide AIDS epidemic. While almost all cases in the United States involved men, in Africa, where large numbers of cases were also occurring, the ratio of men to women was almost one-to-one. The reasons for this phenomenon are still not clear, but plausible explanations do exist. (See Chapter 3.) In the early days of the disease among women in the U.S. who had AIDS, it was not known for certain if some acquired it from heterosexual intercourse. Neither was HIV transmission *from* women proven.

In the March 15, 1985, issue of *The Journal of the American Medical Association*, Dr. Robert Redfield and co-workers reported 5 cases of AIDS in the spouses of 7 males with AIDS. Other reports of such transmission were reported within months by Redfield and others. These studies established heterosexual transmission where previous studies had shown the presence of HIV in semen and vaginal secretions, but not actual male-female or female-male transmission. (With these findings, it is amazing that in most states, AIDS is still neither classified nor managed as a sexually transmitted disease.)

These studies did not receive much publicity, but to some of the public it was becoming apparent that the AIDS issue just might affect them more directly than they had originally thought. The next news event concerning AIDS increased this perception.

Public Awareness Increases

By the end of June 1985, AIDS had exceeded 6,000 cases. While those in public health had been alarmed for several years, the general public was not sure what this epidemic was all about. The large majority of victims were homosexuals, and 90 percent of the population remained strongly averse to such behavior. Thus, AIDS seemed to pose no threat to the general population.

Then, on July 23, 1985, the news leaked out that Rock Hudson had AIDS, and subsequently, his homosexual liaisons became known. On October 2, 1985, Hudson died after a futile attempt at treatment in Paris. This news provided a new perspective for the public. This patient was no obscure person with AIDS. Hudson was a famous actor who had mostly played "good guys," honored the family, and upheld other ideals. If he was a practicing homosexual, how many other "good guys" (famous or not) were also homosexuals? *Who else* might manifest this disease?

Indeed, painful fruit has been reaped. While homosexual activity can be kept discreet, AIDS cannot. Many wives' and parents' first knowledge of their husbands' or sons' homosexuality was the appearance of AIDS. While many homosexuals have "come out of the closet," most have not. In this way AIDS has not only claimed lives, it has destroyed families physically and psychologically.

Physically, AIDS will probably be transmitted to virtually 100 percent of spouses who have sexual intercourse *regardless* of whether condoms are used or not. Twenty to sixty-five percent of babies born to HIV-infected mothers will develop AIDS.[18] If a child is fortunate enough to avoid AIDS, he will lose both parents to the disease. Psychologically, the family not only has to deal with a terminal illness, but one brought on by (what is usually seen as) detestable behavior.

By the end of 1985, 8631 cases of AIDS had been reported, with a slight increase in the percentage of women with the disease.

The Surgeon General's Report

As the AIDS epidemic increased both in numbers and in the public's consciousness, Dr. C. Everett Koop issued his "Surgeon General's Report on Acquired Immune Deficiency Syndrome," to present the "facts" on AIDS.[19] As a Christian, however, he erred on several crucial, moral principles.

1) He did not say that homosexuality is immoral, extremely unhealthy, and a threat to the stability of any society.

2) He advocated sex education in the schools *beginning in kindergarten*! In this recommendation he ignored the immoral principles that are usually taught in these courses. (The statistics clearly indicate that our sex education programs have paralleled an epidemic of teenage pregnancies and sexually transmitted diseases.)

3) He failed to call for standard public health measures for epidemics, such as contact tracing and more widespread testing for HIV. He chose, instead, to rely on "education" as the only method to stop the disease. This "education" is often entrusted to social liberals and homosexuals who produce materials that not only promote their agenda, but are often the worst sort of pornography.

4) He advocated "safe sex" for homosexuals and heterosexuals, yet this message will probably cause more cases of AIDS than it will prevent, because it will give false assurance of protection. Again, sex education and universal contraception for the past 20 years have only resulted in an *increase* in the "problems" (sexually transmitted diseases and unplanned pregnancies) they were supposed to prevent.

Dr. Koop made other mistakes, but these will suffice for now. The perception by his audiences underscores these errors, as Dr. Koop suddenly became quite popular with the homosexuals and other liberals.

> "Unwittingly, the Reagan administration had produced a certifiable AIDS hero. From one corner of the country to another, AIDS researchers, public health experts, and even *the most militant of gay leaders* hailed the surgeon general"[20] (my emphasis).

Simultaneously, he was (and continues to be) attacked by conservatives for a departure from his commitment to their values. If he had maintained the opposite of the four positions above, likely he would have been run out of Washington. At least, however, he would have been consistent with his Biblical beliefs, *and* he would have presented a more sound public health approach to this epidemic.

Dr. Koop defends himself with the premise that he is a public health officer for *all* the people, not just the conservatives. His failure to understand, however, is critical because it is a misunderstanding of truth. God's values *always* are the best directives for the health of both the individual and the public. *Health cannot be divorced from morality*. For Dr. Koop to believe that somehow he can protect the public from themselves and from others with directives not derived from Biblical truth is (bluntly) to say that his wisdom exceeds God's wisdom.

(This failure occurs too often among Christians, especially those in medicine. We should remember that God's principles are *always* the best principles for physical and spiritual health. To think otherwise is to believe that some truth exists that is higher than God Himself.)

The Surgeon General's Report, however, further increased public awareness that this epidemic was going to have considerable impact on American society -- an impact far beyond the risk of infection.

The Heterosexual Issue Surfaces Again

In March 1988, the "sex researchers," Dr. William H. Masters and Ms. Virginia E. Johnson, published their book, *Crisis: Heterosexual Behavior in the Age of AIDS*. It hit the press like a bombshell! "Officials" had been minimizing the threat of the heterosexual transmission of AIDS. Masters and Johnson's figures showed that 7 percent of women and 5 percent of men with multiple partners were HIV positive.

While the validity of their research was questioned by many other "experts," Masters and Johnson did further raise American consciousness that AIDS was not limited to homosexuals and IV-drug abusers. It is obvious that since their report, heterosexual transmission has had an increasing emphasis in medical and news reports. Also, women have continued to show an increasing proportion of new cases of AIDS. In 1988, they accounted for 10.2 percent of the total. Of these, 29 percent were thought to have been acquired through heterosexual contact.

The "heterosexual threat" remains one of the big "unknowns" of the AIDS epidemic, as I will discuss in my forecasts in Chapter 3.

One Minor and One Major Event

The minor event occurred in November 1987, when my newsletter, *Monthly AIDS Update*, was launched. (In January 1990, its name was changed to *AIDS: Issues and Answers*, and it became bimonthly.) It was then, and now remains, the only periodical on AIDS that is explicitly Christian.

The major event was the public health brochure on AIDS in June 1988. It was the first time that the government had mailed anything to every home in the country. That, my friends, is a major event! Since it contained virtually the same public health information as did the Surgeon General's Report on AIDS, I will not comment further.

The Future

We have arrived back in the present. What will the future of the AIDS epidemic be? Only God knows. I will, however, continue to track it and make some predictions through my newsletter. I do not claim infallibility, but I do have a reasonable track record. (See Chapter 3.) This epidemic will be an exciting, although tragic adventure, as it will have a major impact on the human race around the world.

Notes and References

1. Centers for Disease Control, "*Pneumocystis* Pneumonia," *Morbidity and Mortality Weekly Report*, 30 (June 5, 1981):250-252; Centers for Disease Control, "Kaposi's Sarcoma and *Pneumocystis* Pneumonia Among Homosexual Men -- New York and California," *Morbidity and Mortality Weekly Report*, 30 (July 3, 1981):305-308.

2. Judy M. Ismach, "Health Hazards of Homosexuals," *Medical World News*, 22 (November 23, 1981):56-67.

3. *Ibid.*

4. Rimming is the insertion of the tongue into the anus of another person, a common practice among homosexuals.

5. Catherine Macek, "Acquired Immunodeficiency Syndrome Cause(s) Still Elusive," *The Journal of the American Medical Association*, 248 (September 24, 1982):1423-1431.

6. *Ibid.*, 1423.

7. *Ibid.*, 1425.

8. Randy Shilts, *And the Band Played On*, (New York: St. Martin's Press, 1987), 223. I recommend this book for those who want a *detailed* account of the "AIDS story." It is an excellent chronicle of these events, with insights into the homosexual community. Obviously, I do not endorse all his material, since he is a self-admitted homosexual. 617 pages; $24.95.

9. *Ibid.*, 223.

10. *Ibid.*, 220-223.

11. Many lawsuits have been generated by this failure to guard the blood supply. Most have won little or nothing. In all states except New Jersey, blood banks are protected by "blood shield" statutes that classify blood banks as services, rather than as selling a product. Thus, the blood banks have not had their just due for thousands of transfused HIV infections that could have been prevented.

12. Shilts, 450f.

13. *Ibid.*, 592.

14. *Ibid.*, 592.

15. Dennis L. Breo, "Robert C. Gallo, M.D.," *American Medical News*, 30 (December 4, 1987):3, 21f.

16. Shilts, 593.

17. *Ibid.*, 489-491.

18. The transmission rate from mother to child seems to be geographically dependent. In New York City, the rate is may be as high as 65 percent, while other areas are closer to 20-25 percent.

19. C. Everett Koop, "Surgeon General's Report on Acquired Immune Deficiency Syndrome," *The Journal of the American Medical Association*, 256 (November 28, 1986):2784-2789.

20. Shilts, 588.

CHAPTER 3

How Bad Is This Plague Anyway?

Some believe that AIDS will be the worst plague in human history. When the early statistics were doubling every 6-12 months, this prediction seemed quite real. AIDS differs from previous epidemics, however, because it is almost entirely limited to specific groups of people. It has not spread throughout the general population as did the bubonic plague, Asian flu, polio, and smallpox epidemics of the past. If a person is not in one of the "high risk" groups, then he or she has little to fear from HIV.

It is fascinating that *all "official" estimates have been revised downward.* These revisions include predictions for New York City, estimates of the actual numbers infected with HIV, and future AIDS cases. Initial overestimates resulted mostly from an exaggeration of the numbers of homosexuals in the United States. (See Chapter 5.)

HIV and AIDS: A Spectrum of Diseases

One can quickly get lost in the statistics without a clear understanding of the stages of infection of HIV. HIV infection is best understood as a spectrum. When a person first becomes infected, he may experience a "flu-like" illness within a few weeks. Usually, this episode has nothing about it to alarm the person that something much more significant is happening within his body. Symptoms differ from one person to another but may include a sore throat, muscle aches, fever, rash, and headache. Lymph node swelling may or may not be prominent. If it is, this finding may be the only indication that something other than the "flu" is present.[1] The illness may last a few days or 2-3 weeks, but it resolves without treatment.

Then the virus enters a long, quiet period for several years. (Just how long it may remain quiet is still not known, as this disease has been around only 10 years.) During this time, the infected person experiences his usual health. Inside his body, however, the HIV is slowly destroying his T-cells (white blood cells that assist other white blood cells, the B-lymphocytes, to make antibodies). At some point during this "latent" period, the patient may develop lymph nodes that are quite large, but not necessarily painful or tender. At this stage, the HIV is beginning to compromise the body's defenses.

The T-cells are gradually reduced in number until the person's resistance is overcome, and signs and symptoms appear. These symptoms may be due to "opportunistic" infections; that is, infections that rarely infect people with normal immune systems. Or, symptoms may be due to the HIV itself. Signs and symptoms include thrush (a fungal infection of the mouth), inflammation of the gums, herpes Type I lesions (blisters that are extremely painful), diarrhea, fever and sweats, and severe weight loss (the "wasting syndrome"). Neurologic symptoms such as numbness, muscle dysfunction, and confusion may occur. This stage is frequently called AIDS-Related Complex (ARC). It is not yet AIDS, even though the person may be severely ill and die before progressing to AIDS.

AIDS is the final and severe stage of HIV infection and also consists of "opportunistic" infections. Perhaps the most common is *Pneumocystis carinii* pneumonia (a parasitic infection of the lungs). Other severe infections include toxoplasmosis, various intestinal parasites, generalized fungal infections, and unusual strains of tuberculosis. A rare form of cancer, *Kaposi's sarcoma*, typically affects the skin, but growths may occur on almost any organ in the body. Lymphoma, a type of leukemia, may occur as well. Without treatment (with zidovudine [AZT] or other anti-viral drug), one-half of all patients will die within the first year after the diagnosis of AIDS is made.[2]

AIDS is the only stage of this disease that is required to be reported in every state. (A few states require the reporting of any stage of HIV infection.) Thus, the most accurate numbers to track this epidemic are the reported cases. Remember, however, that some 1 million Americans are infected with HIV, so this "reservoir" must be calculated into any predictions concerning AIDS. It is likely that virtually 100 percent of those with HIV will eventually get AIDS, unless they die of another illness or injury during the latent phase of HIV. (See Chapter 12.)

Before proceeding, it is necessary to know that in August 1987, the CDC broadened the criteria for the diagnosis of AIDS. Thus, statistics before and after that time must be compared with that change in mind. The CDC, however, does continue to separate reported AIDS cases into the pre-1987 criteria and the post-1987 criteria.[3]

How I Have Done on My Predictions

Gene Antonio in his book, *The AIDS Cover-Up?*,[4] first published in 1986 and updated in 1987, predicted that 15 million people in the United States would be infected with HIV by the end of 1990, "even if the present rate of AIDS virus transmission was cut in half" (that is, half its rate at that time). He considered these projections "optimistic."[5] (In fairness to Mr. Antonio, he was making these predictions on fewer statistics than are available today.)

Dr. William Campbell Douglass in his book, *AIDS: The End of a Civilization*, projected that from 10 million to 230 million people in the United States would be infected by the end of 1991.[6] Dr. Douglass did not have the limited vision that Mr. Antonio did, as Dr. Douglass' book was published in 1989.

My first prediction was made in January 1988 and focused on the population groups that were becoming infected with the AIDS virus, primarily homosexuals and IV-drug abusers. I doubted rapid spread into heterosexuals and a continuing rise of cases via blood transfusions. Thus, I concluded that "we can project an upper number of HIV infections at approximately 3 million cases."[7] Since HIV may take 10 or more years after the initial infection to cause AIDS in its victim, most of these 3 million would have developed AIDS by the year 2000.

The Centers for Disease Control does not make predictions beyond 3 years, so to get any futuristic projections, we have to project their numbers further than they are willing to do. They estimate that 1 million Americans are now infected with HIV. Another 40,000 are being infected each year. That rate would amount to 400,000 for the decade of the 1990s, for a total of 1.4 million.

In the summer of 1988, I noticed that reported AIDS cases were beginning to level off, whereas they had previously been accelerating rapidly. As this trend continued, in January 1989 I revised my predictions downward to approximately 30,000 each year for a total of about 500,000 cases of AIDS by the year 2,000, and approximately 1 million infected, but not manifesting AIDS.

So, how have I done? My first prediction was too high, but far more accurate than those of Antonio and Campbell. My second prediction has been too low, as approximately 50,000 will be reported with AIDS for 1990. (My error here was not realizing that the CDC's records reflect the year that the diagnosis of AIDS was *made*, not the year that it was *reported*. Thus, numbers for all prior years continue to grow!)

So, I believe that I have been in the "ballpark," contrary to many other conservatives and Christians who have projected worst-case scenarios. I believe that their error was in discounting numbers from the CDC and other studies because of a distrust of not only those statistics, but of modern science and medicine as a whole. I was more accurate because modern science and statistics are useful but must be interpreted in light of a Biblical worldview.[8]

Future Projections: Populations at Risk

First, AIDS is a widespread disease, but one that affects well-defined populations. Cases outside of these groups are unusual. Second, AIDS is concentrated mostly in large cities. For example, at one time, New York City accounted for almost one-half of *all* AIDS cases in the United States. Even in the latest statistics, New York accounts for almost 19 percent of all AIDS patients. Obviously, these two characteristics are linked.

Homosexuals and IV-drug abusers are more highly concentrated in the large cities than in smaller cities and rural areas (although AIDS is beginning to appear in these places).

Thus, the high prevalence (number of current cases) and incidence (rate of new cases) in these "high-risk" populations should not be projected to the general population. Any consideration of the total number of future AIDS patients must consider how many people are in these categories.

The homosexual population, the largest category of AIDS patients, is also the largest group that could be potentially infected with HIV. From various sources, the best estimates are that 2 percent of the males, or 2.5 million men, in the United States practice homosexuality or bisexuality with any regularity. (See Chapter 5.) The actual number may be smaller. And likely, fewer men will be attracted to this lifestyle because of AIDS. Some studies, however, do show that young homosexuals often ignore any advice that might decrease their chances of getting AIDS. Thus, the numbers of homosexuals may not continue to increase, but new HIV infections will continue in this population, because many continue sexual practices that place them at serious risk for HIV infection.

Another statistic needed for this projection is how many homosexuals will eventually become infected. It is conceivable that one-half (1.25 million) will become infected with HIV. For example, in San Francisco, as many as 50 percent have been found to be infected already. While the rate among homosexuals has been less in other locations and their promiscuity has been decreasing to some extent, an eventual number of 50 percent seems reasonable.

The number of heroin addicts is estimated to be 400,000-600,000, with two-thirds or more living in New York City. Thus, the total number of AIDS cases in this population cannot exceed this number, *even if all become infected*.

Cases that result from blood transfusions will not increase at the same rate as they have in the past. With the ELISA and Western blot tests now being used as screening procedures, the blood supply is much safer than in the past. False negatives and very early HIV infections may still result in potentially infectious transfusions, but new cases that occur even with these tests will be relatively few.[9]

Thus, 1.25 million homosexuals and 0.5 million IV-drug users may eventually become HIV positive. The total number of all other categories combined is not likely to exceed 100,000 (and probably much less). These estimates project an upper number of people infected with HIV at approximately 2 million as a "worst-case scenario" within the next 10-15 years. (More likely, however, the number will not be that high. See discussion later in this chapter.)

Even so, there are three major unknowns. 1) Immoral heterosexual sex does not involve the large numbers of sexual partners that homosexuality does, but there are many more millions who are "sexually active." As the number of cases among heterosexuals increases, there could be an enormous spread of the HIV. I do not think that it will occur, but this number should be carefully watched. A future "second-wave" phenomenon could occur. The lack of the occurrence of large numbers of AIDS cases in the heterosexual population could give a false sense of security that causes a rapid escalation of immoral heterosexual sex and a rapid increase of AIDS cases.

2) The virus may mutate to become more easily contagious. Currently, it is quite fragile *outside of body fluids*. Household bleach effectively destroys it. It could, however, mutate so that it can be transmitted through saliva or respiratory aerosols (coughing), in which case the general public could be at risk. I do not think that this sort of mutation will occur. HIV is a rapidly mutating virus, yet since its discovery it has remained remarkably stable in its infectious nature.

3) Some "critical mass" concentration of viruses could be reached. That is, so many people become infected that the concentration of the HIV reaches a point where anyone could be "inoculated" with sufficient numbers of viral particles and become infected by those who are HIV positive, even without "high-risk" behaviors. This situation is not likely either. There is good evidence that "casual" infections either do not occur or are so rare that they are hidden in other statistics. (See Chapter 9.) If some critical mass does occur, however, the death toll will be on the order of the numbers predicted by Antonio and Douglass.

The Epidemic Nature of Viruses

Most readers are probably familiar with the epidemic nature of Asian "flu." (Many may have actually had it! I have.) While there *is* a "flu season" during the winter months every year, it is not always an epidemic, where 30-50 percent of the population is affected. The pattern is episodic.

This episodic nature of viruses may explain the leveling of AIDS cases over the past several years. That is, an epidemic occurred in the late 1970s and early 1980s, but the virus (for whatever reasons) was not transmitted at nearly the same rates after those early years. A change in behavior by some homosexuals may have limited the spread of the HIV, but this effect was minimal, considering that bathhouses remained open, and studies have shown that only a minority of homosexuals have made any significant change in their behavior because of AIDS.

Based upon this reasoning, two researchers have applied Farr's Law of Epidemics to the spread of AIDS.[10] This law was formulated in 1840 to analyze mortality from smallpox in England and Wales and has undergone some modifications since that time. Other details are more lengthy than I can go into here.

With the application of Farr's Law, these researchers believe that the AIDS epidemic crested in 1988, and that there will be a rapid fall-off of cases in the next few years. Total cases will approximate 200,000 by the year 2000. This projection, however, is limited to adult homosexuals, bisexuals, and IV-drug abusers. The researchers are uncertain about the impact of the new diagnostic criteria for AIDS that the CDC instituted in 1987. They also admit to other limitations of their numbers: "We wish to re-emphasize that this projection is a crude, first approximation."[11]

While I agree with the researchers' design that is based upon the epidemic nature of viruses, their projections are too low. The reported numbers of AIDS cases exceeded 170,000 in March 1991, making their upper limits highly improbable, if not invalid. Nevertheless, AIDS has followed an epidemic pattern of rising numbers and a plateau. It is not likely that the usual rapid downslope of an epidemic (when plotted on a graph) will occur for AIDS, because it has become established in specific patterns of spread after the initial epidemic.

The African, Homosexual, and IV-Drug-Abuser Connection

In Africa, HIV is rampant, and the male:female ratio of AIDS patients is 1:1, while the male:female ratio in the United States is 7.5:1 (see below). Public health officials and others wonder whether the same situation will develop in the United States. An explanation for this phenomenon is that there is some "connection" between the groups (homosexuals and IV-drug abusers) with high prevalence rates and Africans.

> These data demonstrate that the immune systems of African heterosexuals, similar to those of U.S. homosexual men, are in a chronically activated state associated with chronic viral and parasitic antigenic exposure, which may cause them to be particularly susceptible to HIV infection or disease progression.[12]

This conclusion followed a comparison of African patients with AIDS (heterosexuals), U.S. patients with AIDS (homosexuals), African men without AIDS (heterosexuals), U.S. men without AIDS (homosexuals), and U.S. men without AIDS (heterosexuals). The first four groups had a high incidence of cytomegalovirus, Epstein-Barr virus, hepatitis A and B viruses, herpes simplex (Type I) virus, syphilis, and toxoplasmosis. They differed from the fifth group in that they (first four groups) had a "significantly greater prevalence of antibodies to each of these infectious agents."

Thus, diseases that are generally "endemic" for Africans (and many Third World people) are endemic to homosexuals in the United States. Interestingly, IV-drug abusers also have a high prevalence of many of these diseases. These diseases and the altered immune states that result are not commonly found in U.S. heterosexual men and women. Thus, this difference may be one factor that limits the heterosexual spread of HIV. (See below for more discussion on heterosexual spread.)

Changing and Static Patterns of Reported AIDS Cases

Top number in each category is 1981 through August 14, 1987
Bottom number is January 1, 1990 to December 31, 1990[a]

	Adult males (%)[b]	Adult females (%)[b]
Homosexual/bisexual	26,086 (65.1) 23,738 (54.8)	---
IV-drug abuser only	5,152 (12.9) 7,689 (17.7)	1,354 (3.4) 2,329 (5.4)
Both homosexual and IV-drug abuser	2,982 (7.4) 2,295 (5.3)	---
Hemophiliac or other coagulation disorder	356 (0.9) 329 (0.7)	8 (0.02) 11 (0.03)
Heterosexual[c]	735 (1.8) 1,054 (2.4)	797 (2.0) 1,657 (3.8)
Transfusion	543 (1.4) 501 (1.2)	296 (0.7) 365 (0.8)
Undetermined[d]	919 (2.3) 2,061 (4.8)	265 (0.7) 528 (1.2)
Sub-total	36,773 (91.8) 36,667 (86.9)	2,720 (6.8) 4,890 (11.3)
Children (all categories, both sexes)	558 (1.4) 782 (1.8)	
Totals (from above)	40,051 (100) 43,339 (100)	

Total of all AIDS cases from 1981 to December 31, 1990: 161,073
(includes the 2 years not shown above)[e]

Explanations

a. Adapted from Morbidity and Mortality Weekly Report, August 14, 1987 and HIV/AIDS Surveillance, January 1991.

b. Percentage of the totals (40,051 and 43,339).

c. Heterosexual sexual partners of persons with AIDS or at risk for AIDS. This category was formerly divided into U.S.-born and persons from a "high-risk" country. The category now has 7 divisions according to sexual behaviors, country, and IV-drug abuse. All involve sexual exposure to someone with or at high risk for HIV infection.

d. Patients for whom information has not been completed or is unknown. When information can be completed on these patients, they fall roughly into the same percentages as the above categories.

e. Showing the first 6 years and 1990 allows a contrast of changes that would not be as apparent if all years were included.

Current and Past Numbers Contrasted

The table above shows some change in the demography of AIDS cases.[13] The top number in each category represents the cases that were diagnosed in the first 6 years of the epidemic, from 1981-1987. The bottom number represents the cases reported for the calendar year 1990. By placing the numbers in this way, we can see changes that have occurred recently. (Note: The total at the bottom includes the 2 1/4 years from August 14, 1987 to December 31, 1989 that are not shown in the table.)

My first observation is that more cases were reported in 1990 than were reported in those first 6 years combined! Also, since the totals are close, comparisons of percentages in each category are valid.

Although IV-drug abusers now account for a greater proportion of AIDS cases than they did earlier, homosexuals still account for the majority of cases. In terms of raw numbers, homosexuals comprise more than 3 times the number of AIDS cases compared to IV-drug abusers. The male:female ratio of AIDS cases for 1990 was 7.5 to 1, compared to 13.5 to 1 in the first 6 years.

The Heterosexual Risk

The (almost) doubling of the numbers and proportion of women with AIDS reflects *exposure to high-risk males* and is not necessarily an alarming increase in heterosexual transmission. The CDC lists 7 sub-categories under "Heterosexual." Every sub-category reflects exposure to a male with HIV infection or at high-risk for HIV infection.

Heterosexual transmission, apart from these direct types of exposure would appear in the CDC's "No Risk Identified," a sub-category under the more general heading of "Undetermined" (the category listed before the sub-totals in the table). CDC personnel vigorously investigate cases that fall into this category. By the end of 1990, the CDC had initially placed 10,224 cases of AIDS in their "Undetermined" category. Of these, 4,528 have been reclassified to one of the other risk categories. Some 1,135 have died, refused interview, or were lost to follow-up. Another 4,110 are still under investigation.

After this thorough investigation, *a total of 469 cases continue to have "No Risk Identified."* This number is 0.27 percent of the total number of 171,876 AIDS cases that have been reported through March 1991. Thus, even if all these cases represented heterosexual transmission, its occurrence accounts for a very small portion of the AIDS population.

The dangers for heterosexual transmission, however, are real, because one partner rarely knows for sure what the other has done. In spite of their "coming out," it is likely that there are still more clandestine homosexual and bisexual men than those who openly admit their deviance. Further, some inner cities now have such a high prevalence of IV-drug abusers and homosexuals that any immoral sexual liaison is often more likely to result in HIV exposure than not.

The far greater danger for the promiscuous heterosexual community is the severe epidemic of other sexually transmitted diseases, for most of which no cure is available. While these diseases are rarely life-threatening, as AIDS is, they cause a great deal of physical and psychological harm. Further, these may be the means by which HIV becomes more widespread in this group. Skin lesions caused by these STDs provide a portal of entry for HIV into the body. This access through damaged skin is considered another reason (in addition to the "connection" above) that the male-to-female ratio in Africa is 1:1.

Other Observations From the Table

Cases of AIDS infections from blood or blood products (hemophiliacs and transfusion recipients) have remained stable or declined. Almost all cases in this category were infected prior to blood screening for HIV, which was instituted in March 1985. The CDC, however, does admit that 15 people with AIDS have become infected by blood that had been screened for HIV, so the problem is not entirely eliminated.

The number and the proportion of children who have become infected from their mothers has increased. Again, this primarily reflects the inner-city culture of IV-drug abuse and promiscuous sex.

An Increase in 1990

The calendar year of 1988 averaged 2733 cases of AIDS reported each month. In 1989, there were 2918 cases per month, a 6.8 percent increase. In 1990, however, there was an average of 3644 cases per month, a *24.8 percent* increase over 1989. I have no explanation for this increase and have seen nothing in the literature about it. Temporarily, however, that trend lessened from October 1, 1990 to January 31, 1991, with an average of 3001 cases per month reported. I believe that the increase represents more efficient reporting or another statistical aberration, but I will continue to watch this trend and for others' explanations of it.

What Does the Future Hold?

We are watching an event that is unique in human history. This epidemic appeared suddenly, virtually exploded in growth in its early years, and has now become another ongoing infectious disease that is routinely reported to public health officials. But will it continue to follow this predictable course? Probably, it will.

Likely, the numbers presented by the CDC are more accurate than they once were. Their projection is 40,000 new *HIV infections* each year (but remember that AIDS, the *reportable* stage of HIV infection, will not appear until many years later). They predict steadily increasing numbers of *AIDS cases* for the next 3 years to the 58,000-85,000 for 1992.

These numbers are probably too high, even though the CDC has revised their original projections downward by 17 percent. *The cases reported to the CDC have not yet reached predicted levels for any year to date*, even allowing for their 18 percent "adjustment" for cases not reported.

We are reaching a period of time that will probably show some (more or less) level patterns of AIDS cases. Because 800,000 (1 million minus almost 200,000 AIDS cases already reported) are already infected, 5 percent of these manifesting AIDS each year would be 40,000 cases. New infections or an appearance rate greater than 5 percent would increase this number.

Since the CDC has repetitively overestimated their numbers, and all other revisions have been downward, I will go with a lower range of 40,000-50,000 new cases of AIDS each year. These numbers may even decline by 10-20 percent after another 2-3 years, as the downside of the initial explosion curve. Realistically, the only way that dramatic *increases* could occur is for HIV to explode among heterosexuals. I do not believe that this phenomenon will occur. Neither do I believe that the virus will mutate to a more virulent form (but I do not discount that possibility entirely).

There is one other possibility. As I explained above, diseases for reasons known and unknown have periodic epidemics. We could have another epidemic spread of HIV for one of these unknown reasons. Even if that occurs, however, it will affect virtually the same sub-groups as it currently does. Thus, those affected will not change, but their numbers could increase dramatically.

As far as HIV's being an infectious disease, then, we have arrived at a period of time that will likely have few surprises. However, certain battles still rage. There is the homosexual and liberal heterosexual agenda being advanced because of sympathy for AIDS victims. There is the economic cost of "education," research, and medical care. There is the threat of infection from patient to health-care worker *and vice versa*. All these and other issues are addressed elsewhere in this book. Lastly, there is the morbidity and mortality of AIDS victims and their families.

HIV disease with all its associated agendas is like no other. Slowly, the disease has reached a predictable pattern. Slowly, the other issues will reach some stable pattern. As evangelical Christians, however, we must continue to strive to understand the spiritual, social, and political issues that have caused this death and destruction.

Notes and References

1. Infectious mononucleosis or glandular fever commonly presents with enlarged lymph nodes. For almost all other diseases, large (an inch in diameter or larger) lymph nodes is an ominous sign.

2. Jeffery E. Harris, "Improved Short-term Survival of AIDS Patients Initially Diagnosed With *Pneumocystis carinii* Pneumonia, 1984-1987," *The Journal of the American Medical Association*, 263 (January 19, 1990):397-401.

3. The major difference between the two definitions is that the later one *included laboratory testing for HIV* that had not been available when the original definition was developed and placed into effect. Centers for Disease Control, "Revision of the CDC Surveillance Case Definition for Acquired Immunodeficiency Syndrome," *Morbidity and Mortality Weekly Report*, 36 (August 14, 1987).

4. Gene Antonio, *The AIDS Cover-Up?*, (San Francisco: Ignatius Press, 1986), 133-134.

5. *Ibid.*

6. William Campbell Douglass, *AIDS: The End of a Civilization*, (Clay-

ton, Georgia: Valet Publishers, 1989), 55.

7. Ed Payne, "How Bad Is This Plague Anyway?" *Monthly AIDS Update* 2 (January 18, 1988):5.

8. This distinction in my approach is quite important for Christians. Some Christians have adopted virtually *carte blanche* the claims of many unorthodox remedies and preached them as gospel. While I have been critical of modern medicine, it *has* produced a vast body of research that should not be ignored, but interpreted from a Biblical perspective.

9. Through February 28, 1991, the CDC reports 15 people who have become HIV positive in spite of blood screening.

10. Dennis J. Bregman and Alexander D. Langmuir, "Farr's Law Applied to AIDS Projections," *The Journal of the American Medical Association*, 263 (March 16, 1990):1522-1525.

11. *Ibid.*

12. Thomas C. Quinn, Peter Piot, Joseph B. McCormick, *et al.*, *The Journal of the American Medical Association*, 257 (May 15, 1987):2617-2621.

13. The latest comprehensive summary on AIDS, entitled, "HIV Prevalence Estimates and AIDS Case Projections for the United States: Report Based Upon a Workshop" from the CDC is available for $3.00 postpaid from Massachusetts Medical Society, C.S.P.O. Box 9120, Waltham, MA 02254-9120. Ask for Vol. 39 (No. RR-16, November 30, 1990).

CHAPTER 4

God's Judgment, AIDS, and the Church

God's judgment is a complex subject. We can, however, justly deal with it if we briefly review the basic concepts and then apply them to this epidemic of AIDS.

God's actions are both *legislative* and *judicial*. In His legislative role, *He alone determines what is right and wrong*. In His judicial role, He determines those who have been righteous (obeyed His laws) and those who have sinned (disobeyed His laws). Then, He rewards the righteous and punishes the sinner. His rewards are called "remunerative justice," and His punishments are called "retributive justice." (Here, *judgment* is the weighing of decisions, and *justice* is the carrying out of the judgment made.)

Relative to mankind, these roles have several applications. First, Adam was called upon to obey God in the Garden. His sin brought God's judgment upon the entire human race (Genesis 3:14-19; Romans 5:12-21). This judgment included physical suffering and death and spiritual suffering and death. It has been and continues to be a general consensus among evangelical theologians that mankind would not suffer any sickness and would not die if Adam had not sinned. The argument for that position is too long to present here, but I have dealt with it elsewhere.[1]

Thus, in Adam, the entire human race was condemned to physical and spiritual punishment. In this ultimate sense, we are all guilty. *None is entirely innocent of the sicknesses that we experience*. This principle, then, is our first concerning God's judgment and AIDS. In His grace and mercy, He simultaneously promised salvation (Genesis 3:15), so believers would escape the fullness of His wrath both now and in eternity. Judgment, then, also applies to the final judgment, after which, God's offer of grace will end (Hebrews 9:27; Revelation 20:1-15).

In between the Beginning and the End, God may mete out punishment on individuals (I Samuel 31), families (Joshua 7), and nations (Jeremiah 39), because of severe and unrepentant sins. Within these concepts, then, is the question of whether the AIDS epidemic is an example of one of His specific acts to punish individuals and/or groups, specifically homosexuals (66 percent of AIDS patients) and IV-drug abusers (22 percent of AIDS patients).[2]

Why He doesn't punish all humans more often and more broadly is a mystery of His mercy. We all sin grievously (even after conversion), yet most of us experience good health and long life. (I am speaking generally, realizing many exceptions.) There is not always a predictable cause-effect relationship between behavior and punishment. For example, a tornado kills and destroys the property of both the righteous and the unrighteous. Biblically, Jesus warned against this direct association of disease and disaster with personal (John 9:1-3) or group sin (Luke 13:1-9).

Even so, we can clearly recognize the consequences of some sins that directly cause disease. Alcoholism causes liver, brain, heart and other organ degeneration, as well as death on the highways. Closely related to AIDS are the sexually transmitted diseases and broken marriages that accompany sexual intimacies outside of marriage. Still, a one-to-one, cause-effect relationship does not exist in every case. Some escape the diseases related to these sinful activities. Why some suffer and others do not is a mystery that only God can answer. This fact leads us to the related concept of the consequences of sin.

Deism vs. the Immanent God

Traditional, conservative (orthodox) Christianity has opposed the mechanistic, Deistic concept that God wound up the universe (like a clock) and let it go, only to function according to His predetermined natural and spiritual laws. By contrast, God is both personal as well as legislative.

Unfortunately, we evangelicals have subtly become Deistic in our concept of the consequences of sin. Theologians say that God is *immanent*, that is, spiritually present in all the events of history. The Bible is literally full of accounts of His personal involvement. Yet, we speak of consequence as though it were totally automatic and predictable. Perhaps it is His personal involvement that explains the lack of 100 percent correlation of sin and its consequences.

The question arises, then, "How can we know when His personal intention to punish has been carried out?" The answer is that *we can know only by revelation, that is, by His telling us*. I have listed examples above concerning God's dealings with individuals, families, and nations. This answer brings us to an extremely important tenet of orthodoxy: God no longer speaks explicitly on any subject to any man or group of men. He has already spoken in the Bible and threatens severe punishment to those who add to or subtract from His words (Revelation 22:18-19).

I realize that large groups of Christians today claim that God speaks to them. While I do not want to offend them, I believe that they would want me to state what I do believe rather than hedge. I respect their right to believe as they do. The point is a major one for theology in general, but less important to our concern here. Perhaps, some have claimed that God has shown them that He has sent His judgment on homosexuals and IV-drug abusers. Even so, we may be able to agree on the following.

I summarize. 1) God's justice begins with His determination of right and wrong. 2) He has judged the entire human race in Adam. All are guilty in that ultimate sense. All disease is indirectly caused by Adam's sin. 3) He will finally judge mankind at the close of time. 4) In between Adam and the final judgment, He sometimes punishes for severe sins either through the consequences of sin or His intentional act to punish. 5) We know of His personal punishment only when He has told us specifically in the Bible.

Romans 1:18-32 has special application to our discussion.[3] The first step toward sin is always a departure from the truth (v. 18b). This departure was the case in original sin (Genesis

3:1-5). In man's depravity, however, there comes a point where God "gives them over" (Romans 1:26) to their impurity. God's actions here are twofold. First, He removes His restraint from continuing and deepening sins. (Man is never as fully sinful as he could be because of this restraint.) Second, "there is the positive infliction of handing over to that which is wholly alien to and subversive of the revealed good pleasure of God."[4] That is, "they reap for themselves a correspondingly greater toll of retributive vengeance."[5]

This passage clearly says that *homosexuality itself* is God's judgment. This point has been overlooked by many Christians whom I have read on this subject.[6] Thus, the presence of open homosexuality in our society was already a judgment of God, completely apart from the issue of whether AIDS is His judgment. If we focus on AIDS as judgment, we have overlooked an earlier step in the progression that is described in Romans.

AIDS is very likely a further judgment on homosexuals ("receiving in their own persons the due penalty of their error," v. 27, NASB). We cannot say so absolutely, however, for the reason above, that God has not revealed this fact to us infallibly. Even so, it is difficult to imagine a disaster or epidemic that is as certainly God's judgment in these post-Biblical times. Also, such judgment is primarily directed towards homosexuals and IV-drug users as a group and most certainly toward society as a whole (because it supports and defends homosexuality as a "right"). It could not be a judgment against these people as individuals, because they do not all become infected. This reality again points to God's personal discrimination in His judgments.

Some Startling Medical Facts

The HIV has some distinctive characteristics. 1) It is an advanced form of virus that is unusually well-suited to causing progressive disease while evading traditional approaches to therapy and immunization. (See Chapter 13.) 2) This virus is designed by nature (God?) to evade the immune system.[7] 3) Testing for a vaccine is limited by the availability of animals that can be infected with the HIV, a necessary requirement for such research. The only animals available are the chimpanzee and the gibbon ape, both of which are endangered species. In 1988, researchers found that mice could be infected with HIV, although the virus did not cause disease in them. However, serious problems may limit the usefulness of these "mouse models."[8] Even research efforts seem frustrated by Design.

4) AIDS catches the state and other institutions in their false value system. On the one hand, the science of modern medicine and the facts about the spread of AIDS require that society recommend "old-fashioned marriage" (a lifelong commitment to one heterosexual spouse). On the other hand, such a recommendation would reverse the "sexual freedom" that society has espoused for the past few decades. Until now, medical care could "cover up" the diseases that ravaged those who were promiscuous as homosexuals or heterosexuals. (Actually, the cover-up is false, because medicine has been able to do little about the spread and permanent damage of STDs.) At this point, however, medicine can do virtually nothing to treat or prevent AIDS.

The Church and AIDS

> "For the most part, the church is frozen. We [Christians] either fear contracting AIDS through casual contact, are angry with people who sin differently than we do, or say 'our people don't do those things.'"

Thus, Jeff Collins, a former pastor and director of Love and Action, an interdenominational AIDS ministry based in Annapolis, Maryland, describes the church.[9] Is he right? Is he wrong? In a major epidemic such as AIDS, especially one that centers around sinful lifestyles, the church would seem to have a major role indeed. I am afraid, however, that few Christians or others have presented a truly Biblical picture of the church's role in HIV/AIDS.

To cover all possibilities that a church might face is far too complex to attempt here. Thus, I will deal with what likely situations that a church might face.

Biblical Truth and the Honor of Christ

A common expression in the Age of AIDS is, "Sooner or later everyone in the United States will know someone with AIDS." A less common expression, but one directed at the church is, "Every church will face the problem of having someone with AIDS in its midst." Both statements may prove true, but the second is more important than the first. To know someone with AIDS is a personal response, but to have someone with AIDS in the midst of a congregation brings considerable responsibility by the church to witness to Biblical truth, honor Christ, and provide for the safety of its members. These three roles do not conflict with each other. Correctly understood and applied, Biblical truth honors Christ and protects His people.

The approach of the church will differ whether the person with AIDS is an adult or a child and whether he is a member of the congregation or not. The issues are church discipline and safety of members. The subject of church discipline is far too complex to discuss here. Thus, I assume its validity.[10] Its practice, however, is almost unknown among churches today and shows how far most churches have strayed from Biblical standards.

The Adult With AIDS

The adult with AIDS who is simply visiting your church requires no action. Likely, the church leadership will not know that the person has HIV/AIDS. Even if they do, he poses no risk, and as a non-member, is not subject to discipline.

The adult with AIDS who is a member of the church, however, requires oversight by the church leadership, to whom I will refer as elders. (See Hebrews 13:17; I Peter 5:1-4.) The elders must know how the person acquired AIDS. As we saw in the last chapter, relatively few cases occur because of transfusion today. All the other categories involve homosexuality, IV-drug abuse, or heterosexual immorality. These practices are sinful and must be investigated as such by the elders. If the person was infected by a blood transfusion, no action is required, because HIV was acquired in an innocent manner.

If HIV/AIDS was acquired through sin, the elders must determine whether the person is repentant. *It is here that most authors writing about AIDS patients in churches fail to present a complete plan.* If the person is repentant, the elders have several options, depending upon the testimony of the person and other evidence of his spiritual maturity or immaturity. The person may be a new or straying believer who needs nurture and oversight. Or, he may have a pattern of confession -- but -- returning to sin. Thus, according to the facts of their investigation, the elders, as representatives of the church, will determine whether any action by them is needed.

For example, almost all Christians caught in such sins need the benefit of concrete, detailed Biblical counseling to help them structure their minds and their daily lives to avoid temptation and opportunities for sin. And, they need to understand clearly what Biblical guilt and forgiveness are.

Any Christian who is unrepentant for any one of these three sinful practices, however, must be disciplined by the church! *Not because he has HIV*, but for lack of repentance. (In fact, the only sin for which church discipline is needed is unrepentance.) I Corinthians 5 is quite clear in Paul's instruction to the elders there about a case of unrepentant "sexual immorality." "Remove the wicked man from among yourselves" (v. 13).[11]

That is, they are not to fellowship with him. "...I wrote to you not to associate with any so-called brother if he should be an immoral person, or covetous, or and idolater, or a reviler, or a drunkard, or a swindler -- not even to eat with such a one" (v. 11). That means that they should not interact with him as they would normally, but encourage and exhort him to repent. For example, if John (under discipline) calls Harry to play golf, Harry might say, "I would like to play golf with you

John, but you are under church discipline. However, I would be glad to spend that time talking with you about the sin in your life that needs correction."

Christians who say that the church should nurture and show compassion towards members with AIDS who are still practicing those sins by which they became infected have ignored these Biblical injunctions. To preserve the honor of Christ, the church may not tolerate open immorality in its midst. The church is not just a place for people to be ministered to, but a place where believers are to grow in Christ and build each other up. (See Ephesians 4:11-16.)

By contrast, the church may and should minister to those outside of the church who are caught in their sins. "I did not at all mean (not to associate) with the immoral people of this world, or with the covetous and swindlers, or with idolaters; for then you would have to go out of the world" (v. 10). Do you see the beautiful balance presented by this passage? We minister to those outside the church regardless of their sins; we minister to those within the church who demonstrate repentance and growth; but, we do not minister to those who profess to be Christians but live immorally.

Elders must make judgments. "For what have I to do with judging outsiders? Do you not judge those who are within the church?" (v.12)

A complicating factor in church discipline is the anti-discrimination laws against people infected with AIDS. The church that disciplines one of its members with AIDS may face a lawsuit. Discipline administered in the "nurture and admonition of the Lord," however, is not likely to face legal action. Of course, as I said above, no one is put out of the church for a particular sin, but only for failure to repent of it. The distinction must be kept clear. The final consideration is that the elders "must obey God rather than men" (Acts 5:29). (Likely, elders who understand church discipline will not swerve from it merely because of the possibility of legal action.)

As to infecting others within the church, the person with AIDS is more likely *to become infected* with infectious organisms that others carry than he is to infect others. However, the elders will need to ascertain specifically his role(s) in the church. These are too various to cover in detail, but some general direction is possible.

In Chapter 9, considerable detail is given about potential situations in which HIV might be transmitted. The elders should study that chapter *as it applies specifically to the person with AIDS in their fellowship*. If he is a former homosexual, they will also have to ascertain whether he may continue to be infectious from any organisms other than HIV that are common to homosexuals. (See Index for references.) Likely, the elders will need a physician to help them with such considerations.

One situation has already arisen: Should a homosexual "support" group be allowed to meet in the church?[12] If the participants are practicing homosexuals, then they do pose a risk of infecting others with organisms common to themselves, if they use bathroom, kitchen, and other facilities. While one church may find that risk acceptable (or provide special housekeeping services) in order to minister to homosexuals, another church may choose to protect its members.

(Note: As churches encounter specific problems, they should write me at Covenant Enterprises. In this way, I can accumulate cases that may be addressed more specifically in my newsletter, *AIDS: Issues and Answers*, or a future edition of this book.)

The Child With AIDS

The child with AIDS will have acquired it innocent of personal sins (although the elders may need to inquire about possible sin by his mother or father, if the child was infected *in utero*). Thus, the church's concern is for the safety of the child and the congregation.

In Chapter 9, I cover possible infectious routes, so those guidelines should be adequate without repeating them here. Basically, children must be protected from the "body fluids" of other children with HIV/AIDS. For example, it would be foolish to allow a child who has HIV and has bitten other children to play in a nursery. It would be foolish to allow an HIV-infected child with diarrhea to stay in a nursery with other children. I do not take the position that these children are without risk to others.

While the risk of infection in these ways is infinitesimal, it *is* present, and AIDS is almost certainly a fatal disease. If it is reasonable for mothers to protect their children from known cases of the "flu," is it not reasonable for mothers to protect their children from the chance infection of a fatal disease?

Confidentiality and AIDS Patients

In a congregation, should the names of patients with AIDS be kept confidential? Yes, *confidentiality should be maintained as far as is Biblical.*[13] The elders, however, should know about anyone who has HIV/AIDS, because they have those responsibilities that I have outlined. However, HIV/AIDS is still a disease that stirs people's fears and concerns. Soon, the fact that someone in the church has AIDS will begin to be whispered and gossiped about.[14] When the elders become aware that this spread is taking place, the matter must be brought before the whole congregation. Thus, the truth will be known and rumors and distortions prevented. (Consider: Leprosy and other infectious diseases were not kept secret in either the Old or the New Testament.)

The Church's Responsibility to Minister

What obligation does your church have to minister to persons with AIDS? Simply, no more or less obligation than to anyone else. Many Christians have made too strong a call for the church to minister in this area. While the numbers of AIDS patients are considerable, they are only a fraction of those patients with severe and terminal heart disease and cancer. Why should a church be obligated to minister to AIDS patients more than to patients with other diseases?

There is the possibility of wrong motives here. Would such preferential treatment be given to AIDS patients if it were not for the liberal-generated sympathy for homosexuals who account for most AIDS patients? If AIDS were a disease entirely divorced from homosexuality, would it receive the legal and political protection, as well as federal funding, that it now receives? I think not.

Christians have been caught twice-deceived here. First, they have been called to respond equally in ministry *without discernment to AIDS patients who are repentant or unrepentant* (above). Second, they have been called to minister to what has been largely a sin-generated disease. If we are to speak of deserving people, who rates higher: the innocent (cancer and heart disease patients) or the guilty (AIDS patients)?

Now -- I am not saying that AIDS patients, including homosexuals and IV-drug abusers, should not be ministered to. I *am* saying that there is *nothing* about them that makes a ministry to them a higher priority than other diseased patients.

Some elders may determine that their congregations are called to a special ministry to AIDS patients. Fine. Commendable. Biblical! But, let's not have a clarion call towards AIDS patients that denigrates the hardships of patients with other diseases. Further, let's be sure that we denounce the sin of homosexuality, IV-drug abuse, and heterosexual immorality as we minister to AIDS patients. We must be careful not to advance the homosexual agenda at the same time that we are extending God's mercy.

Other Issues

I am not convinced that churches need "education" programs on AIDS and "sexuality." Certainly, the elders must be informed to oversee situations that might arise with AIDS patients. They may want to develop a formal policy towards those with AIDS, but it will have to be flexible enough to allow for a variety of situations. They may want to make printed materials available to their members.

I see no reason for special "sex ed" classes, however. Any true church will consistently and periodically teach that God has reserved sexual intimacy for heterosexual marriage only. HIV/AIDS is just one more disease that proves the value of that truth. Sex education is the responsibility of parents. That responsibility should not be usurped by the church or the state, whether parents are faithful to that duty or not. The church is to teach parents who are then to teach their children.

Steps to Consider for Personal Action

We have seen that no one is innocent in the ultimate sense, and as members of our society and the human race, we are all guilty. Further, the church has probably done less than it should have in preventing this epidemic. Some action at this point, however, is possible. I suggest four responses by God's people.

1. We should repent, as members of the church and of the society that has allowed such open and flagrant immorality.

2. We must witness of God's saving grace to the primary groups affected by this epidemic.

3. We should consider what our involvement should be with AIDS patients. Some of us will be called to care for them; others will not. What is most needed is a program to care for the increasing thousands who will acquire AIDS -- in a health-care system that cannot effectively manage this increased load.

4. Homosexuality must be fought vigorously. The Bible is clear that homosexuality is far down the ladder of degradation and in no manner is acceptable to God. It is also destructive of a society in many ways, and quite possibly it is a greater threat than abortion. (See Chapter 5.)

God's judgments between the Beginning and the End are primarily judgments to stimulate people to "turn from their wicked ways." His people should repent and work vigorously in those tasks to which God calls them in this crisis. Those outside of Him should also repent and call upon His provision of mercy in Jesus Christ.

Notes and References

1. Franklin E. Payne, *Biblical/Medical Ethics*, (Milford, Michigan: Mott Media, 1985), 81-83.

2. Centers for Disease Control, *HIV/AIDS Surveillance*, (April 1991), 10.

3. John Murray, *The New International Commentary on the New Testament: The Epistle to the Romans*, (Grand Rapids: Wm. B. Eerdmans Publishing Company, 1968), 34-53. This is one of the greatest commentaries ever written on Romans. Readers are encouraged to review the section on these verses as one of the best descriptions of God's judgment to be found anywhere.

4. *Ibid.*, 44.

5. *Ibid.*

6. Indeed, I overlooked it myself. One of my reviewers pointed it out to me.

7. Warner C. Greene, "The Molecular Biology of Human Immunodeficiency Virus Type I Infection," *The New England Journal of Medicine* 324 (January 31, 1991):308-317. This is a comprehensive article that contains the latest scientific information on the AIDS virus itself.

8. Jean Marx, "Concerns Raised About Mouse Models for AIDS," *Science* 247(February 16, 1990):809.

9. Alice Lawson Cox, "AIDS: What's a Church to Do?," *Moody Monthly* (May 1991):22, 24.

10. Jay E. Adams, *Handbook of Church Discipline*, (Grand Rapids: Zondervan Publishing House, 1986); Daniel E. Wray, *Biblical Church Discipline*, (Carlisle, Pennsylvania: Banner of Truth Trust, 1978); Roger Wagner, "Counseling and Church Discipline - Parts I-IV," *Journal of Pastoral Practice*, 6 (No. 1, 2, 3, 4), 1983), 21-30, 25-34, 33-41.

11. Quoted passages are from the NASB.

12. Support groups often violate Biblical principles. In many situations, refusal to such groups may be more necessary on spiritual than physical grounds. See Jay E. Adams, *The Christian Counselor's Manual*, (Grand Rapids: Baker Book House, 1973), 154-158.

13. Confidentiality must be reconsidered by the church that would follow Biblical practices. It is clear that some things must be "told to the church" (Matthew 18:17). That "telling" is assumed by I Corinthians 5:11, else how will others know "not to associate ... not even to eat with such a one?" See Adams, *Handbook of Church Discipline*, pp. 30-33.

14. Gossip, spreading rumors, and other forms of "behind-the-scenes" talking is unbiblical (James 3:1-18). That sin of the congregation may need to be addressed by the elders, as well as their management of the person with AIDS.

CHAPTER 5

AIDS and Homosexuality Are Symptoms: The Actual Disease Is Our Worldview

We must be careful not to confuse the symptom (AIDS) with the real disease or its cause (a worldview).[1] Symptoms are those disturbances that the patient experiences and then describes to his physician. What he experiences, however, is not the disease. For example, a headache may be caused by a brain tumor or muscle tension. It may also be purely psychosomatic without any physical cause.

What is a worldview? Formally, it is the system of beliefs that explains the actions of all living and non-living things. It may be worked out in considerable detail or it may involve only vague notions. It is personal and individual because no two people agree on every point. Yet, it may share varying degrees of common ground with a formal system of beliefs such as orthodox Christianity or the Humanist Manifesto II. Everyone has a worldview, although most people have not been systematic or comprehensive in their construction of the details of their own worldview. If you want to know with considerable accuracy what you believe, then simply watch what you do, what you think, and what you say. God has made us in such a way that we cannot avoid living in a way that is consistent with our worldview (that is, our personal belief system).

Unfortunately, religions, as worldviews, have been placed into a separate category in our society. I prefer to define religion as every individual's belief system. Thus, religion and worldview should be treated as synonyms. More progress might be made for the proper place of religion in politics and in society if religion were re-defined as "personal belief" rather than a belief in some designated "religion." The atheist may be as fervently religious as the fundamental Christian. As evidence of this religious bent, note the occurrence of such words and concepts as "faith," "belief," and "hope" in Humanist Manifesto II. Secular Humanism should be called "religious" humanism. (By way of interest, the Supreme Court officially listed Secular Humanism as a religion in *Torasco v. Watkins*, 367 U.S. 488, 1961.)

AIDS has occurred within the worldview that accepts (even promotes) homosexuality, heterosexual immorality, and other departures from traditional Christian morality. While AIDS *could have* occurred without this worldview, it *did not*. Sexually transmitted diseases (STDs) have exploded in kind and in number over the last twenty years. AIDS is the latest and the worst in this explosion. Without a change in people's behavior, we can expect other STDs, possibly as severe as AIDS (or worse).

The Biblical Worldview

We must not dissociate the spiritual realm from the physical realm. The Bible clearly states that the physical realm is predicated upon the spiritual realm, not the spiritual upon the physical.

> "By faith we understand that the worlds were prepared by the word of God, so that what is seen was not made out of things which are visible" (Hebrews 11:3, NASB).

> "And He [Jesus Christ] ... upholds all things by the word of His power" (Hebrews 1:3, NASB).

Those who do not believe in the supernatural would not believe this relationship of the natural predicated upon the supernatural. Those who believe in the supernatural, but do not believe in an all-powerful Person, might believe something about things being made out of that which is invisible. Only the

Muslim, Jewish and Christian faiths, however, make the universe "personal." Unfortunately, even with a clear revelation and emphasis on a "personal" faith, Christians often leave the Person out of considerations of nature, or specifically, to our interest, disease.

"... The wages of sin is death ..." (Romans 6:23, NASB). AIDS, STDs, cirrhosis of the liver, lung cancer and other behavior-related diseases show that this verse applies not only to the spiritual realm, but to the physical realm as well.

> "Do not be deceived, God is not mocked; for whatever a man sows, this he will also reap. For the one who sows to his own flesh shall from the flesh reap corruption, but the one who sows to the Spirit shall from the Spirit reap eternal life" (Galatians 6:7-8, NASB).

Not only is the cause-effect relationship of sin and disease ("corruption") present here, but also the cause-effect of "sowing" and "reaping." What is reaped is a multiple of what is sown. One seed produces multiple fruit. Thus, the effects of sin (sexual promiscuity) are reaped in multiples (STDs).

Morality and Medicine

In a real sense, physicians have been accomplices in, if not a contributing cause of, the AIDS epidemic. First, a major portion of our time for the past twenty years has been devoted to the prevention of the effects of sexual promiscuity. We have given contraceptives to reduce the risk of an unwanted pregnancy and antibiotics to treat STDs, with virtually no warning of the risks.

But, we have lied to our patients and to our public. We have lied by statement and by implication that we could avoid these consequences. Can we admit now that we have failed? Only someone *both* morally and medically blind could fail to see that (even apart from AIDS) STDs are worse today than ever before. Today ... after twenty years of more "scientific" medicine than past generations could have dreamed possible. Contraceptives have failed, as well, because we choose to abort

1.5 million babies each year when they (contraceptives) have not been effective, in spite of extremely widespread promotion and use.

Second, physicians have not spoken against the decision of the American Psychiatric Association to make homosexuality legitimate, that is, an alternative lifestyle. The diseases that are rampant in this sub-group are enough to condemn this lifestyle, if physicians were not already committed to its moral position within their worldview. (See later in this chapter.)

All these "facts" only demonstrate that without morality, medicine will aid and abet in the *cause* of more disease than it will ever cure. Today, it is not even necessary to bring in "religious" principles. The medical facts about STDs are striking and real.[2] Will we stop lying to our patients and to our public? Will the profession stop lying to itself?

I think not. You see, a religious view spawns hope. As long as medicine understands itself to be an amoral endeavor, it will continue to hope. But ... it will leave a trail of mutilated bodies and the dead in its philosophical wake. If the ability of "scientific" medicine to solve the problem of other STDs is any indication, AIDS will not be solved, because it is caused by one of the most complex viruses known. Physicians are perpetuators of a morality that is based upon a humanist worldview. They will continue to pour fuel on the very fire that they are trying to put out.

Even the former Surgeon General, Dr. C. Everett Koop, is blind to this fueling. He is grossly inconsistent. He has suggested condoms as one prong of the "attack" on AIDS, but he has not suggested in his attack on tobacco that the risk of cancer of the lung be reduced by filtered cigarettes. Somehow he expects a change in behavior from smokers (who he says are addicted), but not from the fornicators and adulterers (who he has not said are addicted).

The Solution: A Comprehensive Worldview

Christians are facing an increasing number of battles that include abortion, pornography, anti-Christian movies, infanticide, school-based clinics, and sex education in public schools.

We are fighting a "way that seems right unto man, but the end thereof is death." As we fight, however, we must also build a comprehensive worldview. For example, apart from the obvious issues of abortion, homosexuality, infanticide and euthanasia, the practice of medicine has escaped much critical review by Christians.

As I have pointed out repeatedly in many publications, the role of government in medicine must be re-evaluated. In fact, *every* aspect of modern medicine must come under Biblical scrutiny. We cannot settle for patchwork. We must have a comprehensive plan for the whole system. All the pieces have not yet fallen into place, but we are moving in that direction.

The *Journal of Biblical Ethics in Medicine* tackles all these issues. Although I am not its editor, I am its "founding father" and continue on its Board of Governors. It is a publication that is absolutely necessary for anyone who would develop a truly Biblical worldview in medicine.[3]

Pluralism Does Not Work Over the Long Term

The social and political process of our times is pluralism. On the surface it appears ideal, because all groups have input into a matter and a vote is taken to determine policy and direction. Pluralism itself, however, is based upon its own worldview that there is enough agreement among competing systems to formulate "good" for society. It also relies upon the "goodness" of men to be impartial and not take advantage of the power that they wield.

A better description of the situation has been stated by Harry Blamires. We are engaged in "a gigantic battle between good and evil that splits the universe."[4] What we have seen in this century is a gradual replacement of Christian values with non-Christian values. As is now apparent, the intended goal of the non-Christians is at least the complete neutralization of Christians, and at worst, the destruction of Christians.

This situation has occurred for at least four major reasons. First, Christians have not had a comprehensive worldview. Second, the Christian's nature is fertile soil for the dialectic destruction of values. By our nature we are willing to be long-suffering (tolerant) of others. We understand the sinfulness of men and their wretched plight. So we tolerate a position that is maybe only slightly different from our own. But the dialectic continues. We tolerate a little more and a little more. Suddenly, we realize that we are miles from where we should be. Then, change is extremely difficult (e.g., abortion).

Third, we have not realized that the intended goal of every non-Christian system is the destruction of Christianity. This intention can be seen in every nation in the history of the world where Christianity was not the dominant system. Only the complex political system and a lingering consciousness of Christian values have prevented an earlier takeover in the United States. We have reached a point where evangelical Christians have little power and are increasingly being denied their constitutional freedoms. Persecution is only a short distance away.

Fourth, we have confused personal tolerance with social tolerance. As individuals, we are to be friendly and charitable to all people (except in self-defense). In society, however, this tolerance ends where Biblical commands are disobeyed, and the life, liberty, or property[5] of another is infringed upon.

Homosexuality is a representative example. The Bible clearly condemns it; therefore, its practice should be illegal and not tolerated by society. There is, however, a balancing principle. The home is sacrosanct. Without incriminating evidence, authorities should not enter people's homes to investigate whether they are practicing homosexuals. Hidden homosexuality is tolerated because a far greater evil would be the loss of the privacy of the home.

So a Biblical society is an intolerant society at the same time that it is the most tolerant of societies. It allows great freedoms of its people. Those freedoms are protected by the punishment of those evils not Biblically permitted.

A comprehensive, Biblical plan for society is greatly needed. Hindsight is better than foresight, so the current situation may not have been preventable. As we consider homosexuality below, however, we will see the cause and effect of Biblical morality and health and *vice versa* of Biblical immorality and severe illness.[6]

Homosexuality: Medical, Social, and Biblical Views

Two landmark ethical decisions were made in 1973. First, the Supreme Court decided *Roe v. Wade*, making abortion in the United States legal at any stage of pregnancy and subsequently resulting in the deaths of almost 30 million unborn children. Second, the American Psychiatric Association decided that homosexuality was not sexually deviant behavior.

Most Christians did not see the implications of *Roe v. Wade* and were slow to respond to that heinous situation. Now, millions are mobilized to stop abortions. Likewise, most Christians do not seem to have grasped the heinous nature of homosexuality. I confess that until I began to investigate the AIDS epidemic, I was one of those. The case can easily be made that homosexuality is as much a threat to the physical health and social stability of a society as abortion.

There is a certain order to my presentation in this chapter. The medical problems alone ought to convince anyone that homosexuality should be strictly limited in society and certainly not promoted. The societal and criminal problems add more weight. Finally, the Biblical argument strictly prohibits tolerance of open homosexuality.

Lesbians fall under the general category of homosexuals. I will not discuss them, however, due to space limitations and their relative insignificance in the transmission of AIDS. In general, they are fewer in number than homosexuals and account for fewer of the problems that follow. My omission, however, should not be construed to minimize the sinfulness of their condition or the social harm that it causes.

How Many Homosexuals?

Any statistics on the numbers of homosexuals in the United States are "best guesses." If Alfred Kinsey's statistics are still applicable (and there is serious question as to their having *any* validity), then 10 percent are "more or less exclusively homosexual."[7] Other estimates in 1962 and 1971 suggested 1-2 percent and 2-3 percent, respectively. A poll of the Playboy Foundation in 1972 found 1 percent. Paul Cameron conducted a survey that showed 1-2 percent. A 1988 survey by the National Opinion Research Center found 2.8 percent had exclusively male partners.[8]

From these statistics, one may conclude that, *at most*, 4 percent of males are exclusively homosexual. With a total male population in the United States of 120 million, homosexuals would number 4.8 million. Another 1-2 percent may be bisexual. Surveys consistently have a 20-25 percent non-response rate, so the actual number remains unknown. My personal belief from these studies and from the progression of the AIDS epidemic in the United States is that the number is closer to 1-2 percent.

Medical Problems

AIDS. Obviously, the biggest current problem among homosexuals is AIDS. For the 12 months ending March 31, 1991, homosexuals (including those who abuse IV drugs) have accounted for *73 percent of all AIDS cases in adults*. Actually, they accounted for a much higher percentage because they directly or indirectly contributed to the cases in all other categories. While one cannot prove that homosexuals caused the initial infections with the HIV, a strong case can be made that their promiscuity caused the subsequent epidemic.

Hepatitis.[9] Hepatitis B is the most virulent form of hepatitis, with over 20,000 cases each year. Hepatitis A is the most prevalent and accounts for more than 30,000 cases, while Non A, Non B and Unspecified hepatitis cases account for another 5,000. The total is almost 60,000 cases of hepatitis each year. More than half of all cases of Hepatitis B in one study were homosexuals,[10] who comprise (at most) 2-4 percent of the U. S. population.

In October 1987, the U. S. Department of Labor sent a letter to physicians and industry officials. It stated that 18,000 health-care workers may become infected with Hepatitis B each year. Ten percent will become long-term carriers and may have to give up their profession. *As many as 300 health-care workers may die each year* from this disease or its complications.

Contrast these statistics with the fact that less than 50 health-care workers have been (proven) infected with the HIV from needle-sticks or cuts contaminated by HIV-infected patients, and one recently died. Thus, the threat of AIDS as a statistical risk is considerably less than that of infection with hepatitis B. Nevertheless, once acquired, HIV infection is probably 100 percent fatal, where hepatitis B is not.

Sexually Transmitted Diseases. Homosexuals account for half of the cases of syphilis.[11] A "similar increased risk" exists for gonorrhea, venereal warts, and possibly herpes virus infections.

"*Gay Bowel Syndrome.*" This term is no longer used, but several years ago it was used to describe the intestinal diseases found commonly in homosexuals. Most of these diseases are almost unknown in the general population apart from international travel. They represent various infectious agents, including viruses, bacteria and parasites. In one study of homosexuals, almost half had one or more of these organisms. Another study showed that possibly 6-7 percent of homosexuals with these diseases work as *food handlers in public establishments*! One-half this number had had hepatitis A while they did similar work.

While HIV very likely cannot be transmitted by food handlers, these "gay bowel" diseases can easily be spread by hand-hand and hand-food contact from carriers to customers. Is it legal to screen employees in food establishments for their sexual orientation? Of course not! While there may not be a reason to screen food handlers for HIV, there is every reason from a public health viewpoint to identify homosexuals who apply for these positions.

Social and Criminal Problems

Recruitment. While the reasons for the choice of homosexuality may not be clear, it *is* clear that homosexuality is quite uncommon apart from recruitment of "straights" by practicing homosexuals.[12] In the 1940s, when Kinsey asked 2,000 homosexuals why they were homosexual, only 9 percent felt that they were born that way. Some 38 percent had their first homosexual experiences with other homosexuals, 29 percent mentioned a poor parental relationship, and 15 named "unusual circumstances" ("being a sissy" or "not getting along with other kids").

In 1983, 22 percent claimed to have been "born that way," and now 35 percent make that claim. (One wonders about the etiology of this genetic mutation in men! Would you believe a "mental" mutation?) In other words, even today the large majority do not claim to have been born as homosexuals.

Crimes and Social Aberrance. Many homosexuals and their supporters would like others to believe that homosexuals are harmless citizens who only seek their own and are kind, caring individuals. Many may be, but as a group they are anything but benign.[13] Remembering the 2-4 percent of the male population who may be homosexual, this group commits:

* 25 percent of sexual contacts between elementary school teachers and their pupils

* 22 percent of sexual contacts between secondary teachers and their pupils

* 14 percent of sexual contacts between citizens and police

* 9 percent of sexual contacts in work situations

* 12 percent of sexual contacts between stepparents and children

* 8 percent of sexual contacts by religious workers

* 16 percent of sexual contacts with relatives.

Even in what seems to be an area unrelated to sexual preference, 13-31 percent more gays than male heterosexuals reported traffic tickets, automobile accidents (64 percent more reported 2 or more accidents), and careless driving.

Some 171 percent more gays than heterosexual males have attempted suicide; 40 percent more have committed or attempted homicide; and 49 percent more have had a physical fight within the past year. Two-thirds of the mass murders over a recent 17-year period were committed by homosexuals. Homosexuals have also been implicated in 33-50 percent of all recorded cases of child molestation.

Economic Costs. Does anyone want to assess the economic costs of these medical and social problems *apart* from the staggering cost of AIDS? Can any society afford to support such costly activities?

Their Goal Is Not Equality

While the advances of homosexuals have been made under the banner of civil rights and equal rights, we should understand that equality is not their goal. It is only a smoke screen and slogan for the present social and political milieu. What they want is control and power.

Consider one homosexual's arrogant declarations:[14] "We shall sodomize your sons, emblems of your feeble masculinity, of your shallow dreams and vulgar lies." There follows repeated references to "our children," that is, he considers all children to be the legitimate property of homosexuals. Is that not a brazen seizure of power? "There will be no compromises. We are not middle class weaklings.... Those who oppose us will be exiled.... All churches who condemn us will be closed...." With the previously cited evidence of their antisocial and criminal activities, can such threatening goals be discounted?

Perversion is total. Perversion in one area opens the door to all other perversions, as God has graphically described (below). A perverted person will either drag others down with him or exert totalitarian authority because he has cast aside all reasonable and moral restraints.

A Biblical Perspective

The foregoing should be seen as the fruit of Biblical immorality, not as evidence that homosexuality is immoral. With unbelievers, such arguments are necessary because they will not hear the Biblical argument.

Homosexuality is not the worst of sins. While it is an abomination (Leviticus 18:22), so are many other practices (Deuteronomy 7:26, 29:17; Proverbs 3:32, 8:7; Ezekiel 33:29; Daniel 12:11). Homosexuality is not an unforgivable sin, as evidenced by "such *were* some of you" (I Corinthians 6:11, emphasis added). Also, God was willing to forego the destruction of Sodom (origin of the word "sodomy") if Abraham could find 10 righteous people in the city (Genesis 18:32). (He could not. The corruption of that society was virtually total.) The *only* unforgivable sin is blasphemy of the Holy Spirit (Matthew 12:31, I John 5:7-12), that is, a rejection of His witness that Jesus Christ is the propitiation for man's sins.

Homosexuality *is* a sin that is associated with the bottom rung of the ladder of human degradation and is a judgment of God on a society. Romans 1:18-32 shows a process of degradation. First, men "suppress the truth in unrighteousness" (v. 18) in spite of the fact that "God made it evident to them" (v. 19). They begin to worship idols (v. 23). Then, God "gives them over" (vv. 24, 26). (God's "giving over" is one of His judgments. See Chapter 4.) There follows all manner of evil practices that culminate in "hearty approval" of the same (vv. 28-32). God is saying that such practices are evil, but the "hearty approval" of such practices is the culmination.

We have that culmination today. The homosexual not only receives official protection from his role in the AIDS epidemic, but his immoral behavior is subsidized with tax money. Apart from true repentance and obedience to God's Word, our society is in its last days. With open homosexuality and many other evils, we are on the bottom rung of the ladder. Physicians must begin to point out that homosexuality threatens the health of our entire society, even apart from the AIDS epidemic. Social and political leaders must destroy the myth of the peaceful homosexual. Pastors and Christian leaders must present the Biblical understanding of homosexuality as a perversion and judgment on our society and the need of the homosexual to hear the Gospel. While much of the media and many "officials" support homosexuals, 90 percent of people in the U. S. do not approve of homosexuality. A ground swell of dissent and action is needed.

If our society is to be turned, it will be only by God's help. Conviction of sin and true repentance are the work of the Holy Spirit. A corrupt society will have more crime and immorality than either the government or the Church can withstand. (Most churches today do not even seem to know that they have a responsibility here.) An orderly society is either a society of individuals who are mostly moral in their daily behavior, or it is a totalitarian state. All other states are in transition to one or the other.

Ministries to Homosexuals: A Disclaimer

This chapter should not be interpreted *in any way* as a commentary on Christians who minister to homosexuals. I have focused on the problems, not on homosexuality as an opportunity for Christian ministry. Homosexuals, especially if they have AIDS, have great physical and spiritual needs. They are a legitimate area of ministry for churches and other Christian organizations.

Practical Steps

All Christians should know something about the intentions and methods of homosexuals. At least one of the following should be read.

* Dannemeyer, Congressman William. *Shadow in the Land.* San Francisco: Ignatius Press, 1989.

* Magnuson, Roger J. *Are Gay Rights Right?* Portland: Multnomah, 1990.

Notes and References

1. Readers should be aware that I am using "disease" here in the figurative sense. Too many things have been classified as diseases that do not fall into that category, e.g., alcoholism and drug addiction.

2. Joe McIlhaney, *Sexuality and Sexually Transmitted Diseases* (Baker Book House, 1990), has an excellent review of these medical facts. It is not

explicitly Christian, so it can be used with unbelievers as well as believers.

3. The *Journal of Biblical Ethics in Medicine* is published 4 times each year. To subscribe, send $18.00 to Journal, P. O. Box 13231, Florence, SC 29504-3231.

4. Harry Blamires, *The Christian Mind: How Should a Christian Think?*, (Ann Arbor, Michigan: Servant Books, 1963), 70.

5. Someone has said that the original version of the Declaration of Independence read "life, liberty, and property" rather than "life, liberty, and the pursuit of happiness."

6. My thanks goes to H. Vernon Sattler, a subscriber to *AIDS: Issues and Answers*, who sent me a paper that prompted some ideas presented here.

7. Paul Cameron, "A Case Against Homosexuality," *The Human Life Review*, 4 (Summer 1978): 17-49.

8. R. T. Michael, *et al.*, "Number of Sex Partners and Potential Risk of Sexual Exposure to Human Immunodeficiency Virus," *Morbidity and Mortality Weekly Report*, 37 (September 23, 1988):565-568.

9. Hepatitis A is transmitted almost entirely by improper hand washing after defecation (of those who are infected). While people with the disease may be ill for months, they usually get well without complications. Hepatitis B is transmitted sexually, by blood-contaminated objects, and from mother to unborn child. It is usually a more severe disease than hepatitis A and frequently causes long-term liver damage and sometimes death. Some people remain infectious during this long-term phase. Until the last few years, Non-A, Non-B hepatitis has been a catch-all category but now appears to be caused most commonly by a newly identified "C" virus. Its modes of transmission include all the routes of both A and B. It has a 50 percent incidence of the chronic form. Other possible agents in this Non-A, Non-B category are still being defined. "Unspecified" simply means that the form of hepatitis was not identified when it was reported.

10. Miriam J. Alter, *et al.*, "The Effect of Underreporting on the Apparent Incidence and Epidemiology of Acute Viral Hepatitis," *American Journal of Epidemiology*, 125 (January 1987):133-139.

11. Robert T. Rolfs, "Epidemiology of Primary and Secondary Syphilis in the United States, 1981 Through 1989," *The Journal of the American Medical Association* 264 (September 19, 1990):1432-1437.

12. Paul Cameron, *Exposing the AIDS Scandal*, (Lafayette, Louisiana: Huntington House, Inc., 1988), 152-153.

13. Paul Cameron, "Criminality, Social Disruption, and Homosexuality," Family Research Institute, P. O. Box 2091, Washington, DC 20013. Write for a list of all their publications for statistics concerning homosexuals.

14. Cameron, *Exposing the AIDS Scandal*, 35f.

CHAPTER 6

The Family: The Bible and Tradition

The AIDS epidemic has occurred because of violations of Biblical and traditional morality. That understanding is a basic theme of this book. One violation among many is a breakdown in personal and social commitment to the family. Thus, a review of what God designed the family to be has direct relevance to the spread of AIDS *and to the control of its spread.*

The Bible does not succinctly define "family." From its numerous descriptions, commandments, and prohibitions, however, it is clear what God designed the family to be. Departure from this standard causes weak, fragmented families. Individual members also suffer because each family member is most likely to reach his or her full potential only with the proper nurturing of the family. Society suffers also, since no society is any stronger than its families.

The family has a basis within the Trinity, as two members are simply "Father and Son." Together with the Holy Spirit, They have eternal, perfect fellowship. Each has His own responsibilities, while Each is co-equal with the Others.[1]

These characteristics are present in the Biblical family. The core of the family is the husband and wife. Theirs is the most intimate of earthly relationships. They "leave" their own families while they "cleave" to one another (Genesis 2:24). They give themselves wholly to each other (I Corinthians 7:1-5; Ephesians 5:22-33). Their divorce is described as literally a "tearing of flesh" ("separate" = Greek, *chorizo* -- Matthew 19:6; I Corinthians 7:10-11).

A marriage is a link in an intergenerational chain. While they physically leave their own families, the strong, continuing obligations of husband and wife to their parents is reflected in the Fifth Commandment (Exodus 20:12). Paul warns that failure to care for one's parents is to be "worse than an unbeliever" (I Timothy 5:8). Parents are to provide an inheritance for their children (II Corinthians 12:14). The Messiah was promised through a specific family line (Genesis 49:10).

In the Old Testament, "family" (Hebrew, *mishpachah*) is used almost exclusively to denote blood relatives of one or more generations (e.g., Genesis 10:5; Exodus 6:14; Joshua 7:17). The Greek word (*patria*) in the New Testament reflects this link between generations. It is translated (in the KJV) "lineage" (Luke 2:4), "kindred" (Acts 3:25), and "family" (Ephesians 3:15). The most common designation concerning the family is *oikos*, which may refer to the dwelling in which a family lives (Matthew 2:11), or the household, that is, all those who live together under one roof (John 4:53; Philippians 4:22). The latter included servants who lived there. There is little reference in either Testament to the "nuclear family" -- the common term for the family in American society (see below).

The English word "family" is derived from the Latin *familia*, which originally meant "servant." Thus, "family" and "household" from both their Biblical and English roots are synonyms. The Biblical family or household, however, cannot be separated from its intergenerational connection. This unity existed traditionally in the Western world until the last two decades. (Today by contrast, "family" usually designates "household," *separate from* other generations.)

This unity of generations is *totally dependent* upon the lifelong commitment and sexual relationship of a husband and wife. If that relationship breaks (that is, they divorce), the "family" becomes fragmented, and its identity is obscured, if not lost entirely. Thus, there are strong Biblical sanctions against divorce and against sexual liaisons outside of marriage that preserve this unity and continuity. Divorce is permissible only for sexual immorality (Matthew 19:9) and the desertion of an unbeliever from a believer (I Corinthians 7:10-16).[2] God's intent has always been that a man and woman be married for their lifetimes (Genesis 2:24; Matthew 19:8b). English Common Law (based upon Scripture) made divorce quite difficult and provided for possessions to be inherited by the surviving (former) spouse and/or children. In this way, the generations maintained their continuity of lineage and possessions.

Children are an essential part of that continuity. Without children the family line stops. Therefore, the intention by a husband and wife not to have children is inconsistent with God's plan for marriage. Of course, a couple may not be physically able to have children. Their obligations to each other *and the completeness of their marriage*, however, are not lessened by their childlessness.[3] What is forbidden is *an intent* not to have children.[4]

Thus, Biblically, a family must be seen as intergenerational. It cannot be separated from its whole. The "nuclear family," consisting of a husband, wife and children, could be more accurately called, the "one generation family." The "extended family" (the nuclear family plus close relatives) comes closer to the Biblical concept, with its inclusion of parents and other relatives, somewhat like a clan.

The earthly purpose of the family, then, is its nurture of individuals and preservation of continuity with past and future generations. Husbands and wives contribute to the full potential of one another (Genesis 2:18) and train their children for their roles in life (Ephesians 6:4).

In this intergenerational context, no-fault divorce,[5] sexual immorality, and homosexuality are exposed as serious disruptions for individuals and society. Divorce and remarriage multiplies the number of grandparents, aunts, uncles, and other relatives. Relationships become vague and uncertain, especially for children. Individuals are distanced from past generations and their children even more so. Personal identity and belonging becomes more uncertain. In this context, the dramatic and tragic increase in teenage suicide is no surprise. In fact, all social problems are worsened by this lack of family identity.

Homosexuality is an even greater disruption. The norm for any commitment to a "partner" is far less than that for heterosexual relationships, even without marriage. They can have no children of their "coupling" and are thus totally cut off from future generations. Their lifestyle is so far distant from a true family that it can only be considered an abomination by any reasonable, much less Biblical or traditional, standard.

Thus, AIDS can be seen as one "fruit" of the assault on the family. As God has made the Law of Gravity to be inviolate for those who jump without parachutes, He has also made certain laws about health that prevent the acquisition and transmission of sexually transmitted diseases. With the breakdown of the family comes a breakdown of health. No amount of money or medical care will ever be able to bring healing in this context.

Organized Family Medicine Is Anti-Family

The "official" approach to AIDS carries a strong anti-family bias. By "official," I mean the official position of the leaders of the medical profession, the news media, official government agencies, and elected political leaders. While this approach is usually not overt, and its defenders would likely deny this charge, it is nevertheless true. Such an anti-family position is only consistent with the liberal agenda that predominates in the leadership of the United States.

For example, income tax over the last 30 years has gradually decreased the deduction for children (as a percentage of income) to a small fraction of what it was. Welfare benefits for children are usually predicated on the basis of the absence of a man in the home. Divorce is quick, easy, and legally inexpensive. Home schooling has faced strong legal and social pressures. Pornography laws are lax and rarely enforced. Parents have been dragged into court to defend their use of corporal punishment.

To their shame, physicians have adopted and promoted this anti-family bias. Under a pious pretense of being "non-judgmental," physicians are indoctrinated in their training not to bring morality or religion into the physician-patient relationship. Sadly, the American Academy of Family Physicians is no different in this posture than other specialties.

In 1969, this speciality was created to meet the challenge of comprehensive health care for families. While general practitioners had filled this role for decades, some changes were necessary. With the increasing complexity of medicine, physicians could no longer "do everything." In addition, most general practitioners had only 1-2 years of training beyond medical school. Thus, the post-graduate training period was made a standard 3 years, and the new specialty of Family Physician was begun.

Initially, general practitioners headed most programs, training younger physicians to become both practitioners and teachers of family medicine. Knowing that a large part of all medical practices involves non-physical problems, they added "behavioral scientists" to teach this aspect of patient care. In the majority of programs, these are psychologists. Some, however, are ministers, social workers, psychiatrists, and members of other disciplines.

Unfortunately, family physicians under the influence of these behavioral scientists and a general *avant garde* liberalism in medicine have allowed the family to be re-defined in the image of this philosophy. The family is now a "household" that may include any number of people of a variety of sexual or other commitments to each other (see below). The highest standard of morality is that we, as physicians, continue to be "non-judgmental" toward any and all patients.

"AIDS: A Guide for Survival"

In May 1989, all members of the American Academy of Family Physicians (AAFP) were sent a booklet entitled, "AIDS: A Guide for Survival." It had been "favorably reviewed by both the AAFP's Committee on Health Education and Task Force on HIV/AIDS." The AAFP "was pleased to provide" every member a copy "to help meet our members' needs to educate their patients and their communities about AIDS."

Well, another sort of education was covertly taking place. I will mention only two examples, but they are duplicity at its worst. As you read what follows, keep in mind that such has been officially endorsed by the single medical speciality (supposedly) committed to families.

Monogamy and Sexual Intercourse

In the Glossary of the booklet, monogamy is defined as "The custom of being married to one person." While this definition is inadequate, it is not flagrantly erroneous. In the Summary, however, monogamy is defined as a "One-to-one relationship with someone." Could any example of double-talk or George Orwell's "Newspeak" be any more evident? The Glossary definition is virtually restricted to the legal commitment of a man and woman to each other for life. The Summary definition includes any "relationship" between two people of whatever sex with whatever commitment to each other. Is it too much to ask the AAFP to tell us what they really mean, or has duplicity become their style? (Would you, the reader, want the dosages of your children's medications prescribed with such imprecision?)

The Glossary defines sexual intercourse as "The sexual union of a male and a female, in which the penis is inserted into the vagina." This definition is a good one. In the Summary, however, sexual intercourse is defined as "Vaginal *or* anal sex[6] (emphasis added)." Again, AAFP, which is it? Would the real AAFP please take a stand?

One wonders whether: 1) the AAFP is intentionally trying to assist other forces to change our vocabulary and thus change our standards of morality, or 2) the brochure was not adequately reviewed by the committees in their efforts to discover inconsistencies. If the first approach is true, the AAFP is intentionally undermining its *raison d'etre*. Without the family (as defined traditionally), the Family Physician loses his distinction among other primary care specialties (Pediatrics, Internal Medicine and Gynecology). If the second approach is true, the AAFP needs competent administration.[7]

More Anti-Family Positions

I suspect the first approach is true, because the remainder of this booklet mostly advances the same "education" and "condom" propaganda that has "official" endorsement elsewhere. (I will say that at some points it shows a little more caution than other AIDS material.) Also, the AAFP has failed to stand elsewhere for the family. In the April 1989 issue of the newsletter of the AAFP, an "official" release was announced concerning the rights of privacy between adolescents and their physicians. It stated:

> "When, in the judgment of the physician, the well-being of the adolescent patient would otherwise be jeopardized, it is proper and ethical to protect his patient's confidentiality and withhold information from the parent."

There are two things to note here. 1) The AAFP arrogantly assumes that the authority and the wisdom of the physician exceeds that of the parents. 2) This statement is a clever guise to allow physicians to treat adolescents for sexually transmitted diseases, prescribe any form of birth control, or perform abortions. For example, no physician will do a procedure as minor as ear piercing without parental permission, usually written. But, legally, *in all 50 states*, physicians may evaluate and treat a child *of any age* for these three problems *without parental consent or knowledge*. This statement by the AAFP attempts to make these actions moral, as well as legal.

In the Academy Policy on AAFP Positions, "family" is defined as

> "... A group of individuals with a continuing legal, genetic and/or emotional relationship. Society relies on the family group to provide for the economic and protective needs of individuals, especially children and the elderly."

Could any definition be more vague? Teenagers who are "going steady" qualify for this definition! People in business together also qualify. Homosexuals with any sort of (temporary or longer) commitment also qualify.

Back to the Bible and the Traditional Family?

So, what definition of the family should the AAFP use and defend? I suggest that the family consists of a husband and wife who are legally married to each other (and intend to live their entire lives together) along with one or more children. Simply, the family is the nuclear family as it is usually defined. Such a husband and wife without children are part of a family (their lineage and relatives), but in themselves not a family. Nevertheless, a properly stated AAFP commitment could equally include them.

This definition would not prevent Family Physicians from caring for individuals, even homosexuals, who did not fit it. It would, however, underscore exactly whom Family Physicians were primarily trained to treat (*families*) and foster their continuing support and defense of the basic, most stable unit of society. Strong arguments could be presented that this posture would do far more than anything medically possible to maintain health and prevent disease both psychologically and physically.

Thus, the AAFP, along with so many other individuals and institutions, has failed to defend traditional and Biblical values. Social, psychological and physical deterioration can be the only consequence, if this course continues. The worst consequence, however, would be God's continued judgment upon our nation. (See Chapters 4 and 5.)

Practical Steps

Why am I telling my readers of these perverse positions of my beloved speciality? First, these positions of the AAFP are representative of the trend among professionals toward increasingly liberal positions. Second, I believe that action is necessary, depending upon who you are.

Family Physicians. Read the AIDS booklet for yourself and send a fact-centered letter demanding an apology from the heads of the AAFP. Also, ask for official positions, such as the one on adolescent care, concerning the definition of the family and marriage. Write all the other family physicians that you know to do the same.

Consider resigning from the AAFP, if some action to change this anti-family bias is not soon apparent. Unfortunately, the only influence today seems to be an impact upon the pocketbook. I believe that there are enough physicians in the AAFP who are Christians to have a profound effect, if we all withdrew.

Is withdrawal the moral action to take? Why not work within "their" system to change it? While some may believe that they are called to work in this way, it does not seem to be either historically effective or the Biblical method. If one had complete freedom of his time and plenty of money for travel, some influence on policy might be accomplished.

My experience, however, is that leaders and administrators will politely receive you, maybe create some impotent committee, or place you as the lone voice on a large committee. To me, it is a dead-end street. With dues at $460 per year (1989), it would not take many of us (with only this money) to do a direct mailing of our own to the whole AAFP.

Biblically, we are on precarious ground to remain members. We must wrestle with the meaning of the following passage.

> "Do not be bound together with unbelievers; for what partnership have righteousness and lawlessness, or what fellowship has light with darkness? Or what harmony has Christ with Belial, or what has a believer in common with an unbeliever? Or what agreement has the temple of God with idols? For we are the temple of the living God..." (II Corinthians 6:14-16).

At the same time we should not be iconoclastic, looking for perfection. That is why I remained in the AAFP until 1990. With such actions, however, the time came for me to depart. I did not renew my membership in 1990. I sent the national office my letter of explanation, as I had done several years ago when I resigned from the AMA.

Alternative organizations for physicians to join are Physicians for Moral Responsibility (P. O. Box 98257, Tacoma,

WA 98498-0257) and the Association of American Physicians and Surgeons (1601 N. Tucson Blvd., Suite 9, Tucson, AZ 85716). While these groups are not specifically Christian, they are quite conservative and have many solid Christians as members and leaders.

At some time we will need a specifically Christian organization that understands and is committed to Biblical ethics. (The Christian Medical Society is not sufficiently and consistently Biblical for me to endorse it, although it does show signs of gradual change for the better.) I do not now think that there are sufficient numbers of Biblical physicians to start such an organization. My hope is that the *Journal of Biblical Ethics in Medicine* will build a base sufficient to do so.

Patients of Family Physicians. You can first inform your Family Physician that the AAFP is now anti-family in the ways that I have identified. He is likely unaware of these specific immoralities of his organization. Second, you should ask him to agree not to treat your children without your permission. This request should probably be in writing and signed by him. If he refuses, I would look for another physician. Otherwise, he will not honor your family structure. You may want to explore this position with your Pediatrician also, but I do not know what the official policies of their organizations are.

Pastors. Is this topic something to preach about? Should not your congregation know that they cannot trust their physicians to honor their family authority? Shouldn't they know their Biblical roles as parents? I believe that there are enough evangelical Family Physicians and patients that the AAFP could be influenced over these issues. I do not know about other specialties, but I have been impressed with the number of Family Physicians who are Christians. But then, should not Christians (super)naturally be interested in the family?

I am saddened to write of these developments of my chosen specialty. Within the complexity of modern medicine, I believe there is great need for the Family Physician. He must, however, be a champion of the traditional and Biblically defined *family* and not the advocate of whatever philosophies the prevailing winds may stir up.

Notes and References

1. An adequate discussion of the Trinity is *heavy* theology. I cannot even scratch the surface here, but a discussion of the family is incomplete without knowing its analogy with the Trinity.

2. Jay E. Adams, *Marriage, Divorce, and Remarriage in the Bible*, (Phillipsburg, New Jersey: Presbyterian and Reformed Publishing Company, 1980), 23-75.

3. Franklin E. Payne, Jr., *Making Biblical Decisions*, (Escondido, California: Hosanna Book House, 1989), 15-17.

4. Some variations of this description of the family are adoption and celibacy. Adoption of a child by a family makes him or her a member in full standing within that family. Thus, family lines are not limited to biological lines, although that is God's primary means by which children are to be procreated. In addition, God calls some to (that is, gives the gift of) celibacy (Matthew 19:11-12; I Corinthians 7:7-8).

5. For more information on the family and the implications of "no-fault" divorce, write Strategic Christian Services, 131 Stony Circle, Suite 750, Santa Rosa, CA 95401, for their most recent publications.

6. Anal sex is the virtual identification of homosexuality as legitimate. While a few heterosexuals engage in this aberrancy, anal sex is a typical and common practice of homosexuals.

7. From more recent communications, the AAFP (and the AMA) gives every evidence of having become a true bureaucracy. It responds to members with computer-generated forms and letters. If your problem does not fit a square on one of those forms, the system breaks down. In addition, it has an "official" position that no one is really willing to defend, other than simply, "it exists."

CHAPTER 7

The Family: Pediatric AIDS and Sexual Mores

AIDS in children (Pediatric AIDS = PAIDS) is one of the tragedies of this epidemic. Through March 31, 1991, 2,963 children (under 13 years of age) had been reported with AIDS.[1] These comprise 1.7 percent of the total number of AIDS cases. Of these pediatric cases, 1521 (51.3 percent) have died.

Comparison of 1987 statistics will give some concept of AIDS as a pediatric disease.[2] AIDS has become the 6th leading cause of death among children from 1 to 14 years of age.

Causes of Death in Children (Ages 1-14 Years) - 1987

Accidents	7,119	AIDS	467
Cancer (all kinds)	1,686	Pneumonia and "flu"	293
Congenital anomalies (Birth defects)	1,372	Suicide	251
Homicide	741	Cerebral palsy	245
Heart disease	646	Meningitis	176

The statistics for the other diseases are not likely to change significantly, while PAIDS is increasing. For the 24 months ending March 31, 1991, 1466 cases of PAIDS were reported to the CDC, almost half of the number reported since 1981. Likely, then, PAIDS will soon become one of the five most common causes of deaths in children.

The Situation Worsens

Eighty-four percent of PAIDS are infected by their mothers during pregnancy or the birth process.[3] Another 5 percent have been infected via the blood products that they received for their hemophilia. Nine percent received infected blood transfusions and another 2 percent are "Undetermined."[4] Racial differentials of PAIDS include 53 percent Black, 24 percent Caucasian, and 23 percent Hispanic. The sex distribution is almost even, with 54 percent male and 46 percent female.[5]

PAIDS, then, is mostly a reflection of AIDS in women of childbearing age. More accurately, PAIDS is a reflection of AIDS in female IV-drug abusers, because 72 percent of mother-to-baby transmissions are from mothers who are IV-drug abusers themselves or whose sexual partners are IV-drug abusers. Since these categories are the most rapidly increasing category of AIDS cases in adults, we can expect the numbers of PAIDS cases to increase proportionately.

Pregnancy and HIV Transmission

As many as 1 in 50 babies born in New York City have mothers who are HIV-positive. Overall, 30-65 percent of babies born to these mothers will actually have the infection passed on to them. Outside of New York City, most other PAIDS cases have been reported in New Jersey and Florida. Africa has an even worse problem than this country, however. There, some 400,000 cases of PAIDS since 1981 have occurred among infants and children under 5 years of age. Ninety percent of these have occurred in sub-Saharan Africa.[6]

It takes usually a year or more to know whether babies are actually infected with HIV, because they are born with antibodies from their mothers. Once these antibodies disappear in the first 6-12 months of life, a positive test means the baby has developed his/her own antibodies and is infected. Newer and more sophisticated tests can determine earlier whether HIV is present, but these tests are not yet widely available (and may never be because of their cost).

Surprisingly, HIV in women has little effect on pregnancy

rate or adverse outcomes during pregnancy.[7] Bacterial pneumonia during pregnancy and breech presentations (buttocks delivered first) were the only significant differences between women who were HIV-positive and those who were not. No differences were observed in the frequency of spontaneous or elective abortion, ectopic pregnancy, pre-term delivery, stillbirth, or low-birth-weight infants.

Most children who acquire HIV from their mothers will have symptoms by 2 years of age. The average age of onset is 5 1/2 months, but fevers have been detected as early the first month of life. At the other end of the spectrum are those 6- to 10-year-old children who have no apparent disease, but do have dysfunction of their immune systems when tested. Like adults, most die within 24 months of the onset of AIDS.

Infection-to-onset time differs drastically between children and adults, however. Forty percent of children born with HIV will manifest AIDS by the age of 10 months, whereas the average time to onset of AIDS in adults after infection with HIV is 9-10 years. The median survival time for infants is estimated at 6.5 months, and 19.7 months for older children. Anti-viral drugs, such as AZT, are being tested and may increase these survival times in PAIDS.

The Future and a Practical Suggestion

Dr. Robert Redfield of the Walter Reed Army Institute of Research makes the point that AIDS will increasingly become a family disease with "AIDS orphans." With or without condoms, the spouse who has HIV will eventually infect the other spouse. Depending on the time until the onset of AIDS and its severity when it does occur, the surviving children of these couples will become orphaned. Women who become infected by heterosexual contact with IV-drug abusers "typically" have 2 children at the time that they are diagnosed to have HIV.[8] Children who have become infected *in utero* or during the birth process will die, thus wiping out the entire family. Because not all children will become infected from their mothers, however, one expert has predicted that there will be 75,000 to 80,000 HIV-negative AIDS orphans in the next 7-10 years in

New York City alone.[9]

Without doubt, AIDS is a horrible disease. There are few other diseases (except epidemics of the past) where entire families are vulnerable. While children are not innocent in the ultimate sense of sin and guilt, they *are* guiltless of this disease that devastates their bodies and their families. As AIDS spreads among adults, there will be an increasing number of PAIDS and orphaned children. Perhaps, some Christians would prayerfully consider how they could minister to these victims of sexual immorality and IV-drug abuse, even to adopting them. The risk of the children's infecting other members of the family would be infinitesimal. (See Chapter 9.)

Good Housekeeping

Against Good Homemaking

The following review demonstrates how mainstream America has adopted the mores of the sexual revolution -- and will reap the destruction and death that it engenders.

"Alison's Fight for Life"

In September 1989, *Good Housekeeping* ran the story of a 23-year-old woman (Ali) who, in 1988, was found to have AIDS.[10] It is a poignant account of a tragedy, but one that severely distorts the facts and morals of the situation. The woman's mother (Carol) asks, "How could my beautiful young daughter have this terrible disease?" She reasons in this way.

> "Ali had never done intravenous drugs nor slept with a user nor had she ever had a blood transfusion -- up to now, the ways most female AIDS victims have become infected. And, while Carol knew Ali had become *sexually active* when she was a teenager, she also knew that she wasn't *promiscuous*" (my emphasis).

After learning that she had AIDS, Ali "worried that she might have infected her boyfriends...."

Webster's New Collegiate Dictionary (1977) defines *promiscuous*, as "not restricted to one sexual partner." While the article does not give the exact number of Ali's sexual partners, we know that she had at least three (the one that infected her, and her "boyfriends" since then), and the story implies more than that. Yet, her mother never considered her "promiscuous," and Ali never considered her sexual activity as wrong.

Thus, a major publication that has "good" in its name and has stood as a sort of norm for "good" things is promoting the evil agenda of the "sexual revolution," both in its failure to denounce sexual activity outside of marriage and in its advocacy of the redefinition of "promiscuous."

"AIDS ... Can Happen to Anyone"

In sharing their story with a New York newspaper, "They [this family] hoped that by talking frankly about Ali's illness, they could convince others that AIDS can, in fact, happen to anyone --'not just drug addicts and homosexuals.'"

This statement is nothing more than a lie, at least as far as what was meant. Technically, anyone can get AIDS in the rare, rare, rare instance that "anyone" has a transfusion with HIV-infected blood. But, "anyone" who is not sexually promiscuous (according to *Webster*) or does not abuse IV-drugs is not going to "get" AIDS.

As she strives "to promote a better understanding of the disease among the general public," Ali "urges all sexually active students to use condoms" (the same precaution the CDC recommends). In other words, she advocates "safe sex." Why doesn't she urge people to avoid all sexually transmitted diseases by avoiding sexual activity outside of marriage? Why doesn't she say that all other sex is "unsafe sex"? The Good Housekeeping "Seal of Approval" should be placed upon sexual continence outside of marriage and fidelity within it, not upon condoms for sexual license (what God calls *fornication*).

The Prevailing Attitude

In many ways, this article is more disturbing than the propaganda put out by the former Surgeon General, public health officials, the medical literature, and the news media. Ali's story is a portrait of "mainstream" America: well-to-do parents who want the "good life" for their children. The good life includes "sexual activity" but not promiscuity (as it has been newly defined!). It appears that only a few "fundamentalists" take the position that AIDS and other diseases represent moral violations and not random disease ("can happen to anyone").

Ali's "good life" has ended. Neither she nor her parents can see that she has "sown the wind" and "reaped the whirlwind." Worse, she issues a warning that is not only false, but one that is more likely to *increase* AIDS (and other STDs) among young heterosexuals than to decrease it. Even worse, it appears that "America" has also bought such lies. I recall a song of almost 3 decades ago that has the question, "How many deaths does it take 'til we know -- that too many people have died?" Apparently, no number of deaths will convince those who would leave morality and religion out of social and cultural issues.

Notes and References

1. Centers for Disease Control, *HIV/AIDS Surveillance Report*, April 1991, 8.

2. I have extrapolated these statistics from the *HIV/AIDS Surveillance Report* (p. 13) listed above and *CA-Cancer Journal for Clinicians* 41 (January-February 1991):34. Such statistics lag 4 years behind the actual year for which the statistics are compiled.

3. Centers for Disease Control, 8.

4. See page 34 for the explanation of this category of AIDS patients, as used by the Centers for Disease Control.

5. James L. Fletcher, "Human Immunodeficiency Virus and the Fetus," *Journal of the American Board of Family Practice* 3 (July-September 1990):181-192. This review article is a comprehensive resource for those who want more information on PAIDS.

6. No author. "Pediatric Cases Spur Hike in WHO [World Health Organization] AIDS Estimates," *Medical World News*, 33 (October 19, 1990):4.

7. Peter A. Selwyn, "Prospective Study of Human Immunodeficiency Virus Infection and Pregnancy Outcomes in Intravenous Drug Users," *The Journal of the American Medical Association* 261(March 3, 1989):1289-1294.

8. *Medical World News* (July 24, 1989), 43.

9. *Ibid.*

10. Marianne Jacobbi, "Alison's Fight for Life," *Good Housekeeping*, (September 1989) 96, 246-247.

CHAPTER 8

Health-Care Workers and HIV

Physicians and other health-care workers face a challenge with AIDS. Certainly, they have faced other epidemics in the past, yet few, if any, have been as controversial as this one. Physicians frequently differ over methods of treatment in their care of patients, but rarely are heated exchanges provoked as has occurred with HIV-infected patients.

"Unethical to Refuse to Treat HIV-Infected Patients"

These headlines heralded a report of the Council on Ethical and Judicial Affairs of the American Medical Association (AMA).[1] The report reads, "A physician may not ethically refuse to treat a patient whose condition is within the physician's current realm of competence solely because the patient is seropositive," that is, has a positive blood test to HIV. This is an official position of the AMA, because this council has the authority to make policy without the approval of the AMA's House of Delegates (where most official policies are adopted).

Former Surgeon General C. Everett Koop urged medical students to "rediscover" the Hippocratic Oath when he spoke to the American Medical Student Association section at a meeting of the AMA in Atlanta in December 1987. In so doing, he said that physicians "(have) got to be the first line of defense for the human race against the scourge of AIDS."

Thus, the AMA and a Surgeon General have clearly stated certain ethical obligations of physicians toward HIV-infected patients. If you are a health-care worker, do you agree with them, or is there another moral position? Before tackling that question, we will look at the risk for the health-care worker.

The Risk of Infection for Health-Care Workers

As many as 73 health-care workers may have been infected with HIV by patients.[2] The CDC investigates all cases of AIDS that are reported and fall into the "Undetermined" risk category. (See page 46.) Those for whom a risk still cannot be determined are labeled, "No risk identified/other." Of the 469 now in this category, 73 are health-care workers, 39 of whom reported needlesticks and/or mucous membrane exposures "to blood or other body fluids of patients."

The major study of health-care workers exposed to HIV is The Cooperative Needlestick Surveillance Group study. As of July 31, 1988 (the last published report), 1201 health-care workers had been studied.[3] Initially, only workers who had penetrating injuries of their skin by needles or other sharp instruments were included in the study. Later, however, the study was broadened to include exposure to mucous membranes and skin with open wounds. Each exposed worker was tested at six-week, three-month, six-month and one-year intervals. Sixty-three percent were nurses, 14 percent were physicians or medical students, 11 percent were technicians or lab workers, 7 percent were phlebotomists (lab workers who draw blood), 3 percent were respiratory therapists, and 2 percent were members of the housekeeping or maintenance staff.

Eighty percent of the exposures were needle-stick injuries, 8 percent were cuts from sharp objects, 7 percent were contamination of open wounds, and 5 percent were contamination of mucous membranes. *Only 4 workers tested positive*, and all of these were needle-stick injuries. Two were "deep punctures" that occurred during emergency resuscitation of patients. From this data, a "seroprevalence rate" of 0.42 percent was determined. In other words, the statistical risk from a needlestick exposure to HIV is 1 in 250. This figure has become *the official risk estimate* for such exposures. A "deep puncture" almost certainly carries a higher risk.

Some problems exist with this study. First, workers were followed for only one year after exposure. HIV seroconversion[4] has been known to occur later than this period of time. This phenomenon, however, is uncommon and not a serious detraction from the validity of the study.

The frequency of needle-sticks is a second factor. Some occupations more than others, even for the most careful workers, result in injuries that penetrate the skin. Over a lifetime, the health-care worker's risk can be quite high with recurrence of such injuries.

Third, these exposures were self-reported, but some estimates are that only half of all such injuries are reported. This limitation could seriously detract from the study's validity except that health-care workers who acquire HIV would eventually be reported somewhere in the HIV-surveillance system. Numbers significantly larger than those reported by this study could not be hidden for long. The workers themselves would be sure to "get the word out" one way or another.

Health-Care Workers With Risk Behaviors

Through July 10, 1987, a total of 1875 health-care workers (including laboratory workers) had been diagnosed with AIDS.[5] These represented 5.8 percent of all cases of AIDS. They occurred among 6.8 million people in the health-care field or 5.6 percent of the total U.S. working population. Thus, *there is no higher incidence among health-care workers* than in the general population. *Ninety-five percent* of those with AIDS were reported to have a high-risk behavior.

Of 87 health-care workers at the time of this report who had no risk behaviors, information is incomplete on 16, and 38 are still being investigated. *Thus, 33 have no clearly identifiable risk behaviors, including any injury or other exposure to body fluids of AIDS or HIV-infected patients.* These include 5 physicians (of whom 3 are surgeons), 1 dentist, 3 nurses, 9 nursing assistants, 7 housekeeping or maintenance workers, 3 laboratory technicians, 1 therapist, and 4 others who had no contact with patients.

A more recent study of members of the U.S. Army Reserve with medical and health occupations showed that only "never married" men had any increased prevalence or incidence of HIV infection over civilians with nonmedical occupations.[6]

Other Studies

At the National Institutes of Health (NIH) in Bethesda, Maryland, 332 health-care workers with a total 794 needlestick or mucous-membrane exposures to the blood or body fluids of HIV-infected patients have had their blood tested for HIV.[7] None seroconverted. Another study at the University of California of 235 health-care workers has not shown seroconversion in any of them.[8] Neither has a study in the United Kingdom shown seroconversion in 220 health-care workers with similar exposures.[9]

Dental Professionals

Because dental professionals work with saliva (a body fluid known to contain the virus in HIV-infected people) and almost always cause minor gum-line injuries that bleed, they would seem to be one group of health professionals at an increased risk for HIV.

A total of 1309 dental professionals (1132 dentists, 131 hygienists, and 46 assistants) were studied and tested for HIV.[10] None had any behavioral risks for HIV. Ninety-four percent had had accidental skin punctures with instruments that had been used to treat patients. Adherence to procedures designed to prevent infection was infrequent. *Only one professional (a dentist) tested positive for HIV.*

HIV-positive dentists caring for patients has a totally different perspective, however. In Chapter 9, I review the account of one dentist who is known to have infected 5 of his patients.

Good News and Bad News

The good news is that the rate of infection following exposure to HIV is considerably less than that for hepatitis B virus (HBV), which ranges from 6 to 30 percent. Each year 12,000 health-care workers are infected with HBV, 500 to 600 require hospitalization, and about 250 die.[11]

Although far fewer health-care workers are infected with

HIV from patients than with HBV, the numbers of HIV-infected patients are increasing as the infection spreads and the patients begin to live longer with treatment. The worst news is that HIV-infection is probably 100 percent fatal. And -- HIV-infected patients carry other diseases.

Other Diseases of HIV Patients Are the Greater Risk

Cytomegalovirus (CMV) is a common viral infection that produces a "flu syndrome" in adults, usually without complications or long-term effects. In pregnant women, however, the virus can infect the unborn child and cause severe brain damage prior to birth. CMV is an infection common to AIDS patients whose immune systems are compromised by HIV. Nurses who may become pregnant should consider this risk, and they should be tested for antibodies to CMV. Many will have antibodies to CMV, because it is a common infection. If these antibodies are present, then the person is immunized against CMV and is not at risk. If these antibodies are *not* present, then any unborn child is at considerable risk.

Since 88 percent of HIV-infected patients are homosexuals or IV-drug abusers, they carry many other infectious diseases as well. I have already identified the risk from hepatitis B (above) and other diseases that are present in this population (Chapters 3, 5). More recently, tuberculosis has been added to this list, as 8 health-care workers in Florida became infected with tuberculosis on an HIV ward.[12] Further, these tuberculous germs are more virulent than the common form, as they are resistant to many of the antibiotics used against tuberculosis.

Altogether, these diseases pose a greater threat than HIV itself. It is strange that this greater risk is virtually ignored when the "experts" discuss the risk of exposure to HIV-infected patients. I suspect that this avoidance is an oversight and a rather serious one at that, yet it is also related to the usual attempt to downplay the risk for health-care workers.

What Can We Make of This Data?

Perhaps, the first question is, "Can we trust this information?" The great issue for most Christians and other conservatives is how far a "cover-up" extends. One purpose of this book is to show that information can be biased by "experts" and "officials" at all levels concerning HIV and AIDS. All has not been done that could and should have been done to limit the spread of this virus.

There is no question, then, that data can be misrepresented and even falsified. Medical research has had several proven cases of fraud (not related to HIV). To misrepresent or falsify statistics on AIDS, however, would require a conspiracy of considerable dimension. Labs and workers are spread all over the world with numerous people involved in each report.

Some reports have been delayed for several months until a thorough investigation could be made. For example, a researcher in an AIDS laboratory had been infected with HIV for over a year before his case was reported.[13] A National Cancer Institute spokesman reasoned, "...We didn't say anything because we had not isolated the virus." Their concern was whether he acquired the identical strain (he did) that he was working with, or another one.

It is my belief that the epidemiology of AIDS in the medical literature is trustworthy (to the extent medical science in general is trustworthy). In this sense, a "cover-up" has not been perpetrated. The problem has been a failure of "officials" to treat HIV as a sexually transmitted disease with established principles of infection control (contact tracing, partner notification, etc.). Further, these officials have bent over backwards to downplay the role of homosexuals in the spread of AIDS and those diseases endemic to this group.

Are These Exposures Preventable?

The CDC has published their preventive measures to minimize the risks to health-care workers.[14] Many "officials" have argued that HIV-exposure of health-care workers is virtually 100 percent preventable. Their position, however, like so many theories, refuses to face the reality of human frailty, available time, and emergency situations. Dr. Harold O. J. Brown has already addressed some of those arguments for us (Chapter 1).

Health-care workers have been prevented almost entirely from screening patients for HIV in the hospital and other medical settings where such workers might be exposed to the virus. (Dr. Ronald Reed's hospital was the only exception in Pennsylvania. See Chapter 1.) A strong argument can be made that this screening would do more than "universal precautions"[15] to protect health-care workers, because *they could know when to be more careful*, whereas "universal precautions" are just not practical.[16] I predict that such screening will eventually come, as rational measures will eventually be instituted to limit the spread of this disease.

Appendix

Dr. Jane Orient has calculated that the risk of HIV-infection following a needle-stick exposure from an HIV-infected patient is comparable to typically hazardous occupations, such as mining, construction, and work on a Louisiana oil rig! Her calculations may be "too much" for some readers, but they are important for us to understand how she arrived at her conclusions. Thus, I have placed her work in an Appendix, rather than here.

What Are the Moral and Spiritual Responsibilities of Health-Care Workers to Care for HIV-Infected Patients?

First, as far as I am concerned, the AMA and the Hippocratic Oath have absolutely no claim to the allegiance of health-care workers. The AMA has not only agreed with the legality (and immorality) of abortion on demand, but it has filed briefs with the Supreme Court to defend that position. Officially, it is an active champion of abortion.

As to the Hippocratic Oath (apart from the fact that swearing to Apollo and other false deities is anathema for Christians), which version should be followed: the one that includes opposition to abortion, the one that has been modified since *Roe v. Wade* to accommodate abortion, or the one that will be modified to allow euthanasia? Repeatedly, officials of the AMA and others call for physicians to obey the Oath's commitment to the unconditional care of AIDS patients.

The Hippocratic Oath does have commendable principles (and some that are not commendable), but *until such voices demand that the Oath in its original form be followed and abortion eliminated from the practice of medicine*, those who base medical morality upon it have no credibility. Further, the Hippocratic Oath does not say that the physician's obligation to the patient is without regard for his own life. Medical tradition may imply that obligation, but the Hippocratic Oath does not. And to my knowledge, there is no oath that imposes such an unconditional obligation on physicians.

But... What Would God Have Us Do?

The Bible is silent on the specific moral obligations of Christian health-care workers. In fact, the Bible is silent on almost every aspect of the practice of medicine.[17] Roman Catholics would claim one exception in their Apocrypha (Ecclesiasticus 38:1-15). There are, however, Biblical *principles* to be applied here.

First, Christians have a general obligation to care for the diseased and injured, as well as others who are needy (Matthew 25:31-46). The Parable of the Good Samaritan is a supreme example of the depth and degree of this commitment (Luke 10:25-37).

Second, Christians have specific gifts and callings. More in past times than currently, Christians spoke of vocations or "callings." That is, God called them to specific tasks for their life's work. One such calling is that of a health-care worker.

Even so, callings are both general and specific. Generally, Christians are called to be husbands and wives and fathers and mothers (except those who are called to be celibate). They are also called to worship one day in seven, to have fellowship with other believers, and to function in other roles. Among these general roles, marriage and parenting seem to have priority (Ephesians 5:22-33; I Timothy 5:8).

Specifically, some are called to different locations and circumstances. For example, some missionaries are called to risk their lives and those of their families in "regions beyond" (II Corinthians 10:16). Others are called to minister in the United States or other "civilized" locations. Thus, we must consider this diversity in "callings" as we consider the call of health-care workers.

Generally, our call is one of personal sacrifice, even at the risk of danger to ourselves and our families. A specific call, however, may determine the risk that we are willing to take. On the one hand, the husband or wife with dependents may value these roles too highly to assume any increased risk in a role as health-care worker. Thus, he or she may choose not to care for patients who pose this increased risk. On the other hand, some may be called to care specifically for patients with AIDS and other diseases, assuming this increased risk, as some individuals and churches are doing for AIDS patients, and as missionaries have done for centuries.

From a different perspective, *I do not believe that patients have absolute claims on health-care workers*. That is, they cannot abuse themselves in any way that they desire and expect us to attempt to heal and to care for them without regard for our own risk. Some 88 percent of AIDS patients are homosexuals and IV-drug users. The consequences of their "freedom" should not unconditionally obligate others. That is not to say that no one makes mistakes of judgment and sins personally in ways that require medical treatment. It *is* to say that ongoing and entrenched sinful behavior does not have an unconditional obligation on others.

Paul said that those who refuse to work should not eat (II Thessalonians 3:10). He is clear that their disobedience does not obligate others for the simplest of needs. This principle can be applied not only to the danger of HIV to health-care workers, but to other infections as well. Obviously, this principle would not apply to those who are innocent of direct transmission of HIV (hemophiliacs, children, and others).

Of course, there are other considerations: health-care workers' obligations to patients according to written and unwritten contracts, the rights of employers to have certain expectations of health-care employees, the social and contractual obligations of health-care institutions to care for those who pay for these services, and abandonment of patients by physicians and many others. These must all be worked out by each Christian in his or her "vocational" situation. My point here is that patients cannot place unconditional obligations on health-care workers from any consistent moral criterion, most importantly, from Biblical principles.

Notes and References

1. Sari Staver, "Unethical to Refuse to Treat HIV-Infected Patients, AMA Says," *American Medical News* 30 (November 20, 1987):1, 43.

2. Centers for Disease Control, *HIV/AIDS Surveillance Report* (April 1991), 16.

3. Ruthanne Marcus, "Surveillance of Health-Care Workers Exposed to Blood From Patients Infected With the Human Immunodeficiency Virus," *The New England Journal of Medicine* 319 (October 27, 1988):1118-1123.

4. When a person becomes infected with HIV, his body's defenses are activated to fight off and possibly kill the infection. One mechanism is the formation of antibodies to some part of the protein structure of the invading organism. The antibodies then combine with that protein, killing the organism. These antibodies, however, are not always effective, so they may be present without affecting the invading organism. This situation is the case with HIV infections. The antibodies are present, indicating the presence of HIV. Since the antibodies are present in the serum (the clear component of blood), a person without antibodies is "seronegative" and with antibodies is "seropositive." A change from negative to positive is "seroconversion."

5. Centers for Disease Control, "Update: Acquired Immunodeficiency Syndrome and Human Immunodeficiency Virus Infection Among Health-Care Workers," *Morbidity and Mortality Weekly Report*, 37 (April 22, 1988):229-239. At this same rate, there would be approximately 10,000 health-care workers infected with HIV today (mid-1991).

6. David N. Cowan, *et al*, "HIV Infection Among Members of the US Army Reserve Components with Medical and Health Occupations," *The Journal of the American Medical Association*, 265 (June 5, 1991):2826-2830.

7. *Ibid.*

8. *Ibid.*

9. *Ibid.*

10. Robert S. Klein, *et al.*, "Low Occupational Risk of Human Immunodeficiency Virus Infection Among Dental Professionals," *The New England Journal of Medicine*, 318 (January 14, 1988):86-90.

11. Keith Henry and Joseph Thurn, "HIV Infection in Health-Care Workers," *Postgraduate Medicine* 89 (February 15, 1991):30-38. This is a good summary article on this subject.

12. Centers for Disease Control, "Nosocomial Transmission of Multidrug-Resistant Tuberculosis to Health-Care Workers and HIV-Infected Patients in an Urban Hospital - Florida," *Morbidity and Mortality Weekly Report*, 39 (October 12, 1990):718-722.

13. Diane M. Gianelli, "Researcher in AIDS Lab Infected With HIV," *American Medical News* 30 (September 18, 1987):2.

14. Centers for Disease Control, "Guidelines for Prevention of Transmission of Human Immunodeficiency Virus and Hepatitis B Virus to Health-Care Workers," *Morbidity and Mortality Weekly Report* 38 (Supplement 6, June 23, 1989):1-37.

15. Universal precautions are the measures recommended by the CDC for all health-care workers *with every patient* to avoid exposure to infectious agents, such as HIV and hepatitis B. While health-care workers should take reasonable precautions with all patients, universal precautions makes the care of most patients burdensome when they pose only a minimal and easily acceptable risk for health-care workers.

16. Centers for Disease Control, "Recommendations for Prevention of HIV Transmission in Health-Care Settings," *Morbidity and Mortality Weekly Report* 36 (August 21, 1987, No. 2S).

17. Franklin E. Payne, *Biblical/Medical Ethics*, (Milford, Michigan: Mott Media, 1985):101-125.

CHAPTER 9

Casual Infection: The Risk to the Rest of Us

Since the public has known about the AIDS threat, those who do not practice "risk behaviors" have been concerned about the risk of their becoming infected with HIV. Thus, we shall look at the likelihood of other routes of infection, such as mosquitoes and human bites, as well as the risk of "casual" contact with HIV-infected patients and those who have AIDS. This information will be especially helpful to those who minister to AIDS patients.

From other discussions in this book, it should be apparent that I do not take the "official" position on any medical matter, including possible routes of HIV transmission from one person to another. Thus, what I say should not be immediately discounted just because I cite medical studies and agree almost entirely with the "experts" on the improbability of casual transmission of HIV. I differ with them, however, at some key points, as you will see. The great problem is the misinformation that some well-known Christians and conservatives have disseminated. I have mentioned two such authors (Chapter 3).

Official and Unofficial Risk Behaviors

The Centers for Disease Control classifies all reported AIDS cases into specific transmission categories, as presented in Chapter 3. These can be grouped into: sexual intercourse (homosexual or heterosexual), transfusion of whole blood or certain blood products, and mother to unborn child. Although rare, a fourth category of organ transplantation must be added, as several people who received various organs from the same HIV-infected individual have died of AIDS. [1]

The "Other/undetermined" category in the CDC's classification must be considered further. As we have seen, only 469 of 171,876 cases, or 0.27 percent, remain "No risk identified/ other" after further investigation.[2] It is into this category that routes of transmission other than the four above categories would fall. Two conclusions may be drawn about this group. First, if additional routes of infection do occur, they are rare. Second, many of the cases in this category have characteristics that may not be "official" exposures, but are risky nonetheless.

For example, an "unofficial risk" is any sexual intercourse outside of a lifetime of marital fidelity (or in Biblical terms, fornication and adultery), as HIV/AIDS still is not officially classified as an STD by most state public health departments. While the risk at this time may be small, it is not inconsequential. Prostitutes are a particular risk, since in some clinics more than 50 percent test positive for HIV. (Most are also IV-drug abusers or are sexual partners of IV-drug abusers.) This risk is apparent in that 35 percent of the "No risk identified/other" category have had at least one STD, and 34 percent of the men in this category had had "sexual contact" with a prostitute.

Thus, any analysis of the "No risk identified/other" group has too many variables and not enough information to make definitive conclusions about possible cases that may be transmitted by other than "official" routes. More information, however, can be obtained from people who have had considerable exposure to HIV *unrelated to these "risk exposures."*

Evidence From Health-Care Workers

Substantial evidence against casual transmission of HIV has already been presented in the previous chapter. While health-care workers have been infected with HIV by needle-sticks from HIV-infected patients, there are no documented cases of HIV transmission from contact with body fluids. These exposures can be considerable (on a volume basis) from AIDS patients whose physical conditions include copious diarrhea and vomiting, productive coughs, loss of bladder and bowel control, and abusive behavior during periods of disorientation (secondary to dementia). Almost certainly, if HIV transmission were possible via this route, some cases would have already surfaced.

Is Living With AIDS Patients Safe?

Eleven studies have reported on over 700 household or boarding school contacts of both adults and children who have been infected with HIV.[3] Contact has included helping the person to bathe, dress or eat. Eating and drinking utensils and facilities (kitchen, bath and toilet) were shared. These exposures included contact with the saliva or other body secretions of the infected patients (because of the intensive care required by patients with AIDS) and bodily problems that include those listed above. A more recent study in 206 household contacts of AIDS patients also failed to find HIV infection in any of them.[4]

Another study evaluated 89 household contacts of 25 children with HIV infection. "Household members regularly shared items likely to be soiled with blood and body fluids, including toothbrushes, nail clippers, eating utensils, baths, combs, towels, toys, and beds." Further, this study was conducted because "younger children bite, drool, mouth toys, and are incontinent," providing possible HIV transmission to another household member, especially a sibling. All household contacts tested negative to antibodies for HIV. Seventy-nine of them were tested for HIV itself to cover the possibility that any contact was infected but had not yet formed antibodies to HIV (the "window of infectivity").[5] (See Chapter 12.)

The epidemiology of AIDS in Africa also strongly supports this lack of casual transmission. Hundreds of thousands of Africans have AIDS in an environment that is considerably less sanitary than in the United States. It is not infrequent that both parents in a family are infected. Yet, children are not detectable in the epidemiologic pattern of AIDS in Africa except from mother to unborn child.

Should Children With AIDS Attend School?

A distinction should be made between those children who are infected with HIV and those who have AIDS. Most of those with AIDS will not be able to attend school because they will be too sick. Therefore, we are concerned with children who are HIV-positive but have no symptoms or signs of illness.

From the information already presented, these children should be allowed to attend school. (See "Is Fear of AIDS Irrational?" below.) While AIDS is the headline story, children are much more likely to acquire other types of infections at school. Most of these will be the "garden variety" of chicken pox, strep throats and various "flu" viruses. Complications of these "childhood" diseases are rare, but can cause severe illness and death. Yet, few parents ever consider keeping their children out of school to avoid exposure to these diseases. Actually, because these diseases are common, they pose a more serious threat to school children than HIV, which is very uncommon.

That is not to say that there should be no restrictions. For example, a child with HIV who repeatedly bites other children or has vomiting, diarrhea, frequent nosebleeds, fever or other signs of active infection, should not place other children at risk, minimal though it may be. In addition, there may be other situations where the behavior of a particular child (who is HIV-positive) places other children at risk.

Neither is that to say that teachers with HIV or AIDS should be allowed to continue to teach. Those who acquired HIV "innocently" pose no real threat to students. It is wrong, however, for either a known homosexual or a heterosexually immoral person to teach. That situation, however, is only indirectly related to concerns about HIV/AIDS, so it would be inappropriate to address it here.

Breast-Feeding Is a Two-Way Risk

Well-documented cases exist that HIV-infected mothers can infect their breast-feeding infants, and HIV-infected nursing babies can infect their mothers. In Russia, 12 mothers (without other risk factors) have tested positive for HIV over the past 2 years after transmission from their breast-feeding children. These children became infected when they were accidentally injected with a contaminated needle while hospitalized.[6] In the reverse direction, 8 children have been infected while nursing their mothers in unrelated incidents in several countries.[7]

The exact mode of transmission in these cases is unknown, but presumed to be bleeding mouth ulcers in the children and cracked nipples in the mothers. These conditions would allow for blood-blood or saliva-blood exposure for the mother and blood-blood or milk-blood exposure of the nursing child. Since no case of infection via any body fluid other than blood has been proven, the blood-blood route is most likely for both situations.

Why Doesn't Casual Infection Occur?

With the frequency and extent to which many health-care workers and household contacts are exposed to the blood and body fluids of HIV-infected patients, more than a few cases of transmission would seem reasonable. Why, then, doesn't casual infection occur?

1) Blood-blood exposure is almost always required. It would be uncommon for an exposed person to have an open, weeping skin lesion at the site of exposure. Even if a wound were present, it would have to be fresh, because the typical wound will become a thick clot within a few hours and dry within 24 hours.

2) Although all body fluids have been found to contain HIV in infected patients, the concentration of viral particles in most of these fluids is usually low.[8] All infectious processes depend upon the number of infected particles, as well as actual exposure.

3) HIV is not very hardy. While HIV has been reported to survive as long as 15 days on a moist surface, it lives only 3 days when dried.[9] Even so, the "survival" in this experiment was artificial, in that the concentration of the virus used was 100,000 times greater than what usually occurs in the blood of

an HIV-infected person.

4) HIV is not highly infectious. While its routes of transmission have been compared to hepatitis B virus, HIV is 50 times less likely to be transmitted by needle-stick than HBV.[10] This lower rate of transmission underscores the "risk behaviors" that transmit HIV. That is, transmission usually requires repeated exposures of blood-blood contact either by sharing needles in IV-drug abuse or the torn or diseased tissues of one person being exposed to the blood from the torn or diseased tissues of the person infected with HIV.

5) Common household products readily kill HIV. For example, household bleach in a 1:10 dilution, isopropyl (rubbing) alcohol, ethyl alcohol, formaldehyde, Lysol™, hydrogen peroxide, or a temperature of 56°C (133°F) is effective to inactivate HIV within minutes of exposure.[11]

What About Mosquitoes?

Because of this blood-blood requirement, mosquitoes, bed bugs, and other biting/bloodsucking insects seem to be a natural vehicle for HIV transmission. Mosquitoes are known to spread other diseases in this way, such as yellow fever, malaria, and equine encephalitis.

The mosquito uses a small "needle" to penetrate the skin of her (only females "bite") victim and then flies off to do the same to someone else. She could, then, carry HIV-infected blood from one victim to the next. There is serious question, however, whether HIV survives and is able to replicate in these vector hosts.[12]

Mosquito transmission was suspected in Belle Glade, Florida, when a high concentration of AIDS patients was reported there.[13] No child from 2-10 years of age, however, was infected, and neither was anyone over the age of 60 years. Further, antibodies to other infections that are known to be transmitted by mosquitoes did not significantly correlate with seropositivity for HIV. Finally, the area has widespread prostitution and IV-drug abuse.[14]

Africa is an even better example because of the large numbers of AIDS patients in an environment where mosquito transmission of disease is rampant. If mosquitoes transmitted HIV, children would be expected to be infected along with adults, as with other mosquito-borne diseases. But children do not become infected with HIV in any detectable rate other than *in utero* or from HIV-infected blood during a transfusion.

Summary: Absolutes and the Future

While the risk of casual infection with HIV is infinitesimal, it is not zero. The rarity of infection by an unusual route would make its transmission statistically undetectable among the tens of thousands of those acquired by known risk behaviors. Further, unusual situations do occur. Even blood-blood contact can occur in unusual circumstances (below).

The future also may hold some surprises. As the total numbers of AIDS cases increases, the likelihood of exposure increases. For example, HIV transmission by an organ donor was mentioned earlier in this chapter. Infection from a dentist to his patients has occurred (below). In Chicago, two children accidentally stuck themselves with a syringe from a waste container, and during a pelvic exam a physician used a cotton swab that had been previously used on an AIDS patient.[15]

But, life itself is a risk. Far more people will die of traffic accidents than will ever die of AIDS. Far more health-care workers will die of hepatitis B than will die of AIDS (infected by patients). We should not expose ourselves or our children unnecessarily or foolishly, but AIDS is one of the least of our worries, as long as we are sexually moral and do not abuse IV drugs.

Some Unusual Cases of HIV Transmission

The following cases are anecdotes of possible and unusual cases of HIV transmission. *That HIV was transmitted by the route described is not certain.* I present them for readers to realize that absolute assurance with any disease is never possible, and that unusual circumstances may result in the transmission of HIV in spite of assurances.

HIV Transmission in a Bus Accident.[16] In December 1987, a 32-year-old, single male was traveling in Central Africa when the omnibus in which he was riding went over an embankment. He received multiple cuts over his arms, legs, chest, and back. At least 5 injured and bleeding passengers were lying on top of him. He was certain that two of them dripped blood onto him. It was several minutes before he was able to free himself. Two weeks later he ran a fever, and he thought it was due to an infected wound that had not healed.

Two and one-half months later, he underwent various tests to exclude diseases that he might have acquired on his trip. Testing for HIV was included because of his blood-blood exposure. He tested positive.

Briefly, other possibilities of HIV-exposure were virtually (but not absolutely) eliminated.

HIV Transmission Between Brothers.[17] In 1982, during an open-heart procedure in the first year of life, a male child was infected with HIV. He died of AIDS 3 1/2 years later. When other family members were screened, the boy's brother, 3 years older, tested positive to HIV. All routes of infection were eliminated, except that the older boy had been bitten by his brother 6 months before he died. The mother had seen teeth imprints on the skin, but no bleeding or bruising.

In separate incidents around the world, 16 other people bitten by AIDS patients have remained HIV-negative.[18]

HIV Transmission During Acupuncture. A 17-year-old boy living in Paris tested positive for HIV after a febrile illness and enlarged lymph nodes.[19] All usual routes of transmission of HIV were absent from his medical history. Researchers believed that the most likely route was acupuncture procedures that the boy had undergone for tendinitis secondary to intensive training for rugby.

Other unusual routes for blood-blood transmission have been suggested, but not necessarily reported. These include contact sports injuries, where one player's blood mingles with that of another; "French" kissing, where both partners have bleeding gum disease or mouth ulcers; and oral sex, where lesions may be present in the mouth and on the genitals. Likely, you can conjure up other scenarios where blood-blood contact may occur. Contact with other body fluids is much less likely to transmit HIV, if it is possible at all.

Is Fear of AIDS Irrational?

As we have seen, considerable evidence exists that casual transmission of HIV is rare. Why then does the fear of AIDS cause public demonstrations and hostile acts? Are these fears irrational? While the human mind is much less fathomable than most psychologists (Christian or non-Christian) would admit (Jeremiah 17:9), nevertheless, some reasons for this public fear are likely.

First, the fear of AIDS comes primarily from the public's abhorrence of homosexuality. While the second largest group of AIDS patients, IV-drug abusers, may also be abhorrent, AIDS was initially and remains largely, a disease of homosexuals. To get AIDS is to get a homosexual disease. The overwhelming majority of the American people still abhor homosexuality in spite of the news media and government bombardment of propaganda.

Less important, but still a contribution to this fear, is the fact that AIDS is virtually 100 percent fatal. Getting AIDS is not like getting a cold, pneumonia, or even tuberculosis, which most people survive. The diagnosis of AIDS is a horrible death sentence. Statistically, however, this fear is irrational. As we have seen, other diseases pose a far greater risk on a statistical basis than HIV infection. In general, the public does not fear these common diseases as they fear AIDS. No one has campaigned to prevent children with measles or the flu from attending school.

"Officials" and government policymakers have aggravated this fear in their attempt to quell it. The public will not accept homosexuality as "an alternative lifestyle" (although this attitude appears to be softening). They know that homosexuals' behaviors are grossly aberrant. If homosexuals did not practice such behaviors, they would not now be dying of AIDS by the thousands. But, the prevailing policy and "educational materials" have promoted (indeed, <u>encouraged</u>) homosexuality. Worse, such education has been forced by law to be presented in public school classrooms. Often, any attempt to allay the public's fear was hypocritical.

David Chilton, a pastor and author, tells of a televised program in San Francisco in 1987 that was intended to reassure people about the safety of being around AIDS patients.[20] The audience was invited to call in to the panel of medical experts with their questions, so he did. His request was to have someone on the panel share a glass of water with an AIDS victim. Such a demonstration would be far more powerful than just words of reassurance and statistics! But, the call monitors refused to present his proposal to the panel. In such subtle and not-so-subtle ways, the hypocrisy of the "experts and officials" continues. They are quite willing for the public and health-care workers to take risks, but they themselves are not willing to do so.

Further, *HIV/AIDS is a politically protected disease.* Exceptions have been made for it that have never been made for any disease transmitted sexually. Clearly, such policy was in deference to homosexuals.

Thus, what at first was public concern about AIDS became distrust. Distrust bred fear that indeed a "cover-up" did exist. The public does not have access to the medical literature or government records. What the government tried to do back-fired and caused an increase in the very problem that it tried to quell.

In the midst of all this propaganda, conservatives and Christians looked to their champion, Surgeon General Dr. C. Everett Koop, for morality and leadership. Instead, they got the same propaganda -- delivered to their own homes via the AIDS booklet sent to every known address in the United States. Dr. Koop could have rallied his people and probably the public as well, but he said he was the Surgeon General and not the "Chaplain General," and that he was the Surgeon General of *all* the people -- not just of conservatives and Christians. He missed his day in history. While he may have been run out of Washington, he would have "stood in the gap" (Ezekiel 22:30) and possibly turned the tide toward a scientific and moral approach to AIDS, rather than the prevailing political agenda.

A Personal Aside

Some may conclude from my reassurances that I am in league with "the establishment," but I believe that my opinions in this book and elsewhere prove otherwise. On some issues, I agree with mainstream opinion, whether secular or Christian. On other issues, I could not disagree more radically. I will not hedge where I believe a radical position is closer to the truth, but neither will I distort the facts just for sensationalism or to sell copy. I also try to keep a reasonably open mind. I am not infallible and have been known to change my mind when confronted with additional facts (Biblical, medical, or otherwise).

My goal is the dissemination of the truth, as best I can understand it from a Biblical and a medical perspective. I realize that the truth is not easily determined. I am not unstudied in the philosophical difficulty of what is and what is not truth. Further, the determination of truth is hampered by our finite and sinful limitations. Within these limits, truth is inevitably influenced by one's worldview. For me, this worldview is based upon clear Biblical principles and my own knowledge and experience in medicine with the input of knowledgeable and thinking Christians.

A Dentist Infects Five of His Patients With the AIDS Virus

It is virtually certain that three patients were infected by their dentist. The story began (publicly) on July 27, 1990, when the Centers for Disease Control, in their major publication, *Morbidity and Mortality Weekly Report (MMWR)*, reported the "possible" transmission of HIV from a dentist to one of his patients.[21] Subsequently, the patient, Kimberly Bergalis, identified herself to the public and was featured as the cover story for *People* magazine, October 22, 1990.

Later, the CDC issued a follow-up report in *MMWR*.[22] All totaled, 5 patients (coded A, B, C, D, E) of this dentist, Dr. David J. Acer, who practiced in Jensen Beach, Florida, were found to test positive for HIV. One patient ("D") had "established risk factors for HIV infection," and another's ("E") "laboratory and epidemiologic investigation has not yet been completed."

How Much More "Proof" Does One Need?

All 5 patients had viral sequencing performed. In this procedure, regions of base-pairs (chemical bonds) of the genetic structure of the HIV were determined. These sequences were then compared to HIV from the dentist, to 7 "controls" (HIV patients randomly selected from within a 90-mile radius of the dentist's practice), and to 21 other "North American isolates."

The average difference between HIV from the dentist and patients A, B, and C was only 3.4 percent, while the average difference between patient D, the control patients, and the North American isolates was 13 percent. *"This degree (96.6 percent) of sequence relatedness has been reported only for multiple HIV strains obtained from a single person or for HIV strains from persons whose infections were epidemiologically linked"* (that is, from persons who had infected each other). The viral sequences from the dentist and patients A, B, and C "were not closely related to the viral sequences from patient D, the controls, or the North American isolates."

"... This investigation strongly suggests that at least three patients of a dentist with AIDS were infected with HIV during their dental care...."[23] That statement is as definite as any that you will ever get from a scientist, especially concerning transmission of HIV. I would upgrade their "strongly suggests" to "as conclusive as science can be concerning the transmission of HIV" and "as conclusive as science is almost anywhere, especially in medicine."

By the scientists' own analysis, there is only 1 chance in 167 random occurrences that HIV sequences from patients A, B, and C would be closer to the sequence from the dentist than to the sequences from the controls.

How Did the Dentist Infect These Patients?

Possible routes of transmission include "multiple opportunities for the dentist to sustain needle-stick injuries or cuts with a sharp instrument," "barrier precautions (rubber gloves, masks, etc.) that were ... not always consistent," and contaminated instruments. "The precise mode ... remains uncertain." All that is to say: It is impossible to determine how he infected his patients.[24]

It Is Time to Confront Your Dentist ... and Others

In many ways, patients have more power than physicians. Patients will not be brought before a hospital or county medical society committee because they asked "insensitive" questions or failed to follow the special exemptions of HIV/AIDS patients. Ask your dentist if he has been tested for HIV. If you are facing surgery, ask if any of the surgeons have HIV. Perhaps, if you are highly suspicious, you could ask for reassurance *in writing*.

More importantly, while in the hospital or doctor's office, observe those who draw blood or handle other "body fluids" and also touch you in any way. Too often, you will find hands or clothes that are contaminated.

You would not be unreasonable if you asked a person who is going to perform a procedure (especially one that will open or penetrate the skin, such as drawing blood, giving an injection, and doing a finger stick) to wash his/her hands in your presence. Then, he/she should wear gloves while doing the procedure. The wrapping for any sharp instrument (needle, lancet, etc.) should be opened in your presence, or in the case of non-disposable instruments, assurance given that the item has been appropriately sterilized (autoclaved, sterile solution, etc.). *Nowhere should you see blood from another patient on the instruments or on the person who does the procedure!*

Admittedly, it is difficult to make these requests, but enough patients acting in these ways will put even more pressure on hospital staffs and other governing bodies to do what they should have been doing in the first place: protecting themselves and their patients, not the homosexual who has committed himself to a life that is inherently self-destructive. It will also make medical personnel more careful, because they know that you are watching them closely.

The ADA Comes Through, and Kim Settles for $1 Million

In a new policy statement, the American Dental Association stated that "HIV-infected dentists should refrain from performing invasive procedures or should disclose their seropositive status."[25]

Kimberly Bergalis, patient "A" above, has won a $1 million settlement against her dentist's insurer.[26] (They got off cheap!)

Both actions are too little, too late. With at least 5,000 "innocent"[27] people dead or manifesting AIDS, the medical and dental professions should only hang their heads in shame for violating their oaths and their own standards of infection control.

Kimberly is a victim of this "politically protected disease." She is dying.

> "Do I blame myself? I sure don't ... I blame Acer and every one of you ... Anyone that knew Dr. Acer was infected and had full-blown AIDS and stood by not doing a ... thing about it. You are all just as guilty as he was.
>
> "I have lived to see my hair fall out, my body lose over 40 pounds, blisters on my sides. I've lived to go through nausea and vomiting, continual night sweats, chronic fevers of 103-104 that don't go away anymore. I have cramping and diarrhea ... I have lived through the tortuous acne that infected my face and neck -- brought on by AZT."[28]

She is a sad testimony to medical and dental professions that violated the first premise of care: "First of all, do no harm."

Notes and References

1. These cases appeared in the news media in May 1991. It seems that the donor had only recently acquired HIV and was murdered before his body could make the antibodies that were tested for at the time of his death in 1985.

2. We have already looked at this category twice and examined its breakdown, pp. 34 and 78. For further analysis, see Kenneth G. Castro, *et al.*, "Investigations of AIDS Patients With No Previously Identified Risk Factors," *The Journal of the American Medical Association* 259 (March 4, 1988):1338-1342; Alan R. Lifson, "Do Alternate Modes for Transmission of Human Immunodeficiency Virus Exist? A Review," *The Journal of the American Medical Association* 259 (March 4, 1988):1353-1356.

3. Lifson, "Do Alternate Modes...," 1353-1356.

4. G. Friedland, *et al.*, "Additional Evidence for Lack of Transmission of HIV Infection by Close Interpersonal (Casual) Contact," *AIDS* 4 (July 1990):639-644.

5. Martha F. Rogers, *et al.*, "Lack of Transmission of Human Immunodeficiency Virus From Infected Children to Their Household Contacts," *Pediatrics*, 85 (February 1990):210-214.

6. Rebecca Voelker, "HIV Tied to Breast-Feeding," *American Medical News*, 33 (July 20, 1990):36.

7. S. K. Hira, *et al.*, "Apparent Vertical Transmission of Human Immunodeficiency Virus Type 1 by Breast-Feeding in Zambia," *The Journal of Pediatrics*, 117 (September 1990):421-424.

8. Jay A. Levy, "The Transmission of AIDS: The Case of the Infected Cell," *The Journal of the American Medical Association*, 259 (May 27, 1989):3037-3038.

9. "Survival of HIV on Environmental Surfaces," *Wisconsin AIDS Update*, (April 1988), 21.

10. Gerald Friedland, "Risk of Transmission of HIV to Home Care and Health-Care Workers," *Journal of the American Academy of Dermatology*, 22 (June 1990):1171-1174.

11. *Ibid.*, 1173.

12. Lifson, "Do Alternate Modes...," 1355.

13. K. G. Castro, *et al.*, "Transmission of HIV in Belle Glade, Florida: Lessons for Other Communities in the United States," *Science* 239 (January 8, 1988):193-197; Centers for Disease Control, "Acquired Immunodeficiency Syndrome (AIDS) in Western Palm Beach County, Florida," *Morbidity and Mortality Weekly Report* 35(October 3, 1986):609-612.

14. Christopher Boyd, "Crisis of AIDS Is Magnified by Small Town's Way of Life," *Chicago Tribune* (June 24, 1991, Section 1):5.

15. *Chicago Tribune*, April 26, 1991, Section 2, p. 6; *Chicago Tribune*, May 18, 1991, Section 1, p. 18)

16. David R. Hill, "HIV Infection Following Motor Vehicle Trauma in Central Africa," *The Journal of the American Medical Association*, 262 (June 9, 1989):3282-3283.

17. Volker Wahn, "Horizontal Transmission of HIV Infection Between Siblings," *Lancet*, 2 (September 20, 1986):694.

18. Lifson, "Do Alternate Modes...," 1353.

19. D. Vittecoq, *et al.*, "Acute HIV Infection After Acupuncture Treatments," *The New England Journal of Medicine* 320 (January 26, 1989):250-251.

20. David Chilton, *Power in the Blood: A Christian Response to AIDS*, (Brentwood, Tennessee: Wolgemuth and Hyatt Publishers, Inc., 1987):26ff.

21. *Centers for Disease Control*, "Possible Transmission of Human Immunodeficiency Virus to a Patient During an Invasive Dental Procedure -- Florida," *Morbidity and Mortality Weekly Report* 39 (July 27, 1990):489-493.

22. Centers for Disease Control, "Update: Transmission of HIV Infection During an Invasive Dental Procedure - Florida," *Morbidity and Mortality Weekly Report*, 40 (January 18, 1991):21-27, 33. In addition to these 3 confirmed patients, 2 more are now known to have been infected with HIV by Dr. Acer.

23. *Ibid.*, 23-24. The reason for the small percentage variation of HIV in the same patient is that HIV mutates rapidly, resulting in several genetically different strains in the same patient!

24. *Ibid.*, 26.

25. No Author. *American Medical News*, January 28, 1991, 2.

26. *The Augusta [Georgia] Chronicle*, January 24, 1991, 2A.

27. By "innocent" patients, I mean those infected by blood transfusions, blood products, and unfaithful spouses. Most could have been prevented by proper blood screening and contact tracing.

28. David Zeman, "AIDS Victim Infected by Dentist Writes About Her Anger, Pain," *Chicago Tribune* (June 23, 1991, Section 1):6.

CHAPTER 10

The Economic and Social Impact of AIDS

AIDS has put to rest forever the notion that whatever "consenting" adults do in private does not affect others. That notion was always a lie, but this plague has made it totally untenable. While we have seen that the threat of infection is not something that most of us will have to worry about, we will be (and have been) impacted economically and socially by this epidemic.

The economic costs are difficult to figure because many aspects of the AIDS epidemic are changing. 1) The future numbers of AIDS cases are not known with certainty. 2) AZT and other antiviral drugs may delay the onset of AIDS in HIV-infected patients and may prolong the lives of AIDS patients. Thus, inpatient and outpatient costs will vary considerably, depending upon how effective or ineffective these treatments are. (Outpatient costs are considerably less than inpatient costs.) Thus, one of the most important figures, the cost of treatment for an HIV-infected person for his lifetime, is not known at this time.

3) The number of asymptomatic, HIV-infected people who will be treated with AZT or other antiviral drugs is not known. Currently, only 10 percent of these people know that they are infected, and fewer than that are on AZT.

So that we can get some perspective, I will assume the numbers and projections of my conclusions in Chapter 3. That is, there are currently 1,000,000 HIV-infected people, with an additional 40,000 being infected each year. There are about 80,000 patients with AIDS (including an estimated 20 percent unreported cases).

The Medical and Social Costs of HIV/AIDS

Personal medical care costs. The direct cost for care for one AIDS patient was estimated in 1986 to be $147,000 over his lifetime (14-18 months) after the diagnosis of AIDS is made. After more AIDS patients have been followed in different locations, this cost has been lowered to $80,000 with a life expectancy of 20 months.[1] Thus, the cost for the care of the current 80,000 patients over their lifespans will be $6.4 billion. Applying this same rate to the 100,000 who have died already, their care has cost almost $10 billion.

The cost of AZT treatment for HIV-infected patients is estimated at $6,000 per patient per year. If one-half of these patients (500,000) are eventually placed on AZT, this cost would be $3 billion *per year*. At the rate that people are coming forward to be tested, even with some evidence that early treatment is effective, it is unlikely that more than half of those who are HIV-infected will ever be identified or treated.

Non-personal costs. These costs include research, education and blood testing. Projections are that these costs will be $1.2 billion this year (1991), with a cumulative cost of $5.5 billion by the end of that year.[2]

Indirect Costs. This figure is one that is often overlooked concerning the cost of disease. It is the lost productivity over a patient's lifetime because of illness and early death. Since the ages of most AIDS patients are 20-40 years, they lose from 25-40 years of productivity. The fact that IV-drug abusers are non-productive is balanced by the estimate that homosexuals have above-average earnings. On these bases, costs will be $49 billion this year, with a cumulative cost of $168 billion since the epidemic began.

This figure for 1991 will represent about 1 percent of the projected Gross National Product for the year. It seems a small percentage until one realizes that the GNP grows only 2-4 percent each year.[3] So, the absence of AIDS patients could mean a 25-50 percent reduction in the growth of the GNP for 1991.

Who Pays?

Medicaid and Medicare. Who pays these big bills for medical expenses? *Everyone pays* -- through taxes and insurance premiums. For example, 21-54 percent of AIDS patients are covered by Medicaid.[4] The larger figure comes from IV-drug abusers concentrated in the Northeast who obviously have no income, as contrasted with homosexuals in San Francisco who are typically employed and privately insured.

Most estimates predict that eventually 40 percent of all AIDS patients will be paid for by Medicaid. I predict that the percent will be even higher, because historically, almost every projection of a federal or state medical payment program has exceeded, if not *greatly* exceeded, initial projections. (See "AIDS and Medical Economics" below.)

Already, special provisions have been legislated to allow patients with AIDS to qualify for Medicaid more easily and rapidly than other applicants. In other words, the AIDS patients are being given preferential treatment. There seems to be the strange notion that the exhaustion of an AIDS patient's estate to pay for his medical care is an injustice that deserves more support than cancer, heart disease, or other "traditional diseases."

Medicare is not severely threatened by AIDS. There are few people with AIDS over 65 years of age, and those who do fit into this category acquired AIDS via blood transfusions. Medicare, however, faces its own financial problems, apart from the problem of AIDS. The addition of AIDS patients will only increase these problems.

Medical insurance. Private insurance plans have paid for 17-55 percent of the costs of AIDS patients, varying from one part of the country to another. This situation is complex. Insurers have faced considerable public pressure to accept all new applicants without screening for AIDS. In some cases they have even faced legislative restrictions from doing so.

One proposal is "risk pooling," whereby all insurance companies within a state contribute to a "pool" to provide medical insurance for those who have been turned down for insurance coverage because they are "bad risks." Nationally, all but one of these plans have lost money in spite of high premiums, large co-payments, and high deductibles. Mario Cuomo, when Governor of New York, proposed legislation that would prohibit AIDS testing in health insurance applicants.

One problem that could develop is that most health insurance is provided through group plans -- usually one's employer. These plans usually "take all comers" (without screening) by virtue of employment. Thus, these plans may eventually feel a greater "crunch" from AIDS than individual plans where screening *does* take place (assuming legislation does not prohibit all screening). Indeed, this trend has begun (below).

Life Insurance. Nowhere has the political protection of AIDS patients been more evident than in life insurance. I remember the night when I was traveling, listening to "Talk-Net," a call-in talk show on personal finances. One caller was inquiring how he could get life insurance in Washington, D.C. The host was incredulous to find out that virtually all carriers were issuing *no* new policies, because they were prohibited from screening for HIV.

The same has subsequently happened in California, and 12 other states have restrictions of some type against screening for those at risk or positive for HIV. Few "innocent" (of HIV) have probably been more affected by this epidemic than people in these areas who have tried to obtain a new life insurance policy.

Insurers, however, to protect the premiums of their customers and their assets, are sometimes able to devise ways to circumvent these restrictions. For example, in California, where they cannot test for HIV, they test for a T-cell subset (the blood cell affected by HIV). It remains to be seen, however, who will win this battle between restrictive legislation and private insurance. The trend is to have private insurers bear more and more of the burden of AIDS-related life and health insurance.

The problem of "adverse selection" is more serious for life insurance than for medical insurance. The latter is eventually limited by the patient's death, but life insurance has virtually no upper limits, if one is willing to pay the premiums. In 1986, one percent of all claims were AIDS-related. Some officials have estimated that an increase to 4-5 percent of all claims could "threaten the benefits of all policy-holders." [5]

This impact is also evident in the sizes of the policies. The average AIDS-related claim in 1986 was $30,500 for individual policies and $27,300 for group policies.[6] By contrast, the average claim for all causes was $7,300 and $13,800, respectively. (Part of this difference may be explained on the basis that a younger population has more life insurance than an older population.)

These figures changed in 1988.[7] The average individual claim for life insurance for a patient who died of AIDS declined to $19,500, but the average claim for group claims increased to $27,300. The decrease in individual claims was attributed to an increase in HIV-testing before policies are written.

Other Effects

Hospitals. Many hospitals are absorbing a considerable portion of the costs of AIDS patients. In 1987, 72 percent of all AIDS patients were treated at public hospitals, 26 percent at private hospitals, and 2 percent at V.A. hospitals.[8] With cutbacks in Medicare, hospitals often have to balance their books by cost-shifting from well-insured patients to those patients for whom they receive inadequate reimbursement because they are indigent or because the third-party payer does not meet the hospital's full charges.

Eventually, most AIDS patients exhaust their personal resources, but all of them will not be covered by Medicaid. Thus, the hospitals have to absorb these costs. The greater the numbers of AIDS patients that a hospital treats, the greater this cost-shifting must be. It is predicted that many inner city hospitals will close because of the huge cost burden that AIDS will be for them.[9]

Large cities. The greatest problems will be faced in urban areas. New York, San Francisco, and Los Angeles together account for 31 percent of *all AIDS patients* in the United States. Other cities account for the majority of other AIDS patients. In New York, the cost of caring for AIDS patients is estimated to be $1-2 billion for 1991, or a cost of $100-200 for each resident. With a smaller population, the cost for each resident of San Francisco will be $350. These cities are already clamoring for the federal government to "come to their rescue" financially.

Large cities have other "fallout" from the HIV epidemic. A person is less likely to get a hospital bed when needed because of the influx of AIDS patients. If admitted, he is more likely to have contact with a patient with AIDS either directly or indirectly as they move through the same testing and treatment areas. While the risk of infection is quite small, it is not zero. (See Chapter 8.) The emotional impact of finding oneself in close proximity to an AIDS patient could be considerable in itself.

Neglect of other medical problems. AIDS funding has gone far beyond its proportion of the total health-care problem in the United States. Funding for AIDS research now exceeds that for cancer and heart disease. By comparison, AIDS affects tens of thousands, but cancer and heart disease affects hundreds of thousands. A ground swell of public opinion, however, is beginning to be voiced as this statistic becomes known. Its efficacy to change the preferential status of HIV/AIDS patients, however, is yet to be measured.

False positives. With newer and more sophisticated tests, the chances for false positives have virtually been eliminated. However, most screening will continue to be done with the ELISA and Western blot tests, which detect antibody, rather than the virus itself. (See Chapter 11.) While the rate of false positives is quite low even with these tests, a low rate can translate into large numbers where mass screening takes place. (See Chapter 11.) After these false positives are reported to the patient, there will still be considerable anxiety over the weeks necessary to run the newer tests. Life and health insurance applications may be postponed indefinitely. Explanations to spouses, family, and others will be difficult at best! Jobs could be jeopardized (in spite of judicial protection).

True positives. For true positives, more problems will occur. "Surprises" will be all too common. Fornication and adultery among Christians, according to recent studies, is not far behind that of the general population. Thus, homosexuality among Christians may be more common than might be predicted, also. An ongoing sexual liaison may be hidden, but HIV positivity will eventually manifest itself! It is rare that HIV infection comes from a "one night stand."[10] (See Chapter 11 for a more complete discussion of true and false positives.)

Geopolitical. There are increasingly reliable reports that AIDS will devastate Africa and other Third World countries. With the predominantly heterosexual spread that is epidemic there, the general population will be more greatly affected than in the United States. For example, the prevalence of HIV positivity among prostitutes approaches 100 percent in some cities in Africa.

The political problems in Africa are as unstable as any in the world. With tens of thousands dying of AIDS, we can only expect more instability. The situation will be ripe for dictatorships, anarchy, violence, and outside manipulation by major powers. Thus, AIDS may well have a major political impact in parts of the world -- even apart from personal suffering.

Summary

The impact of HIV will be felt by the sexually moral to a far greater extent economically and socially than from the frequency of actual infection. It will be costly and may bring about the demise of the Social Security system more quickly than would have otherwise occurred. It will threaten the solvency of health and life insurance programs to the extent that they are restricted from free-market forces.

But, brothers and sisters in Christ, there is reason to hope. Many current systems need to be done away with and more Biblical ones instituted. We must prepare and move toward these challenges.

AIDS and Medical Economics

AIDS epitomizes several crises in Western thought. First, AIDS is a crisis of immorality. Scores of new sexually transmitted diseases did not give pause to the "sexual revolution."

AIDS *did*.

Second, some health-care workers have refused to care for AIDS patients to protect themselves and their families from HIV that they might accidentally acquire from patients. In the history of these caring professions, these servants have rarely refused to care for others, even when their own lives were threatened. Yet, in the face of AIDS, they say that individuals and society do not have the right to indulge appetites to the extent that health-care workers' lives are threatened.

Third, AIDS has exacerbated the crisis in payment for health-care services that has been developing for the past two decades. Thousands of patients with AIDS are flowing into a system that is already severely stressed. As yet, no comprehensive plan has been developed to manage this added burden to the system. To understand this situation, however, we must understand something of the forces that produced this crisis and consider the Biblical principles that apply.

Because of our context, I will have to be brief where a more complete development is really necessary. The *Journal of Biblical Ethics in Medicine*, however, has had several articles that give more information on this subject.[11]

An Historical Perspective

After World War II the costs of hospitalization and surgery came to be considered as an unexpected financial burden on individuals and families. (From today's perspective, however, those costs were quite minimal!) Prior to that time throughout history, medical costs were borne almost entirely by the patient, his family, or charity.

The idea was conceived that risk for these medical expenses could be pooled, such as had been done with fire insurance for homes. Thus, a third party was brought into the relationship between the physician and the patient, and medical insurance was born. It was a nice system for all. Physicians and hospitals were paid more promptly and fully. Patients did not directly face the economic burdens of surgery and hospitalization. Insurance companies had another means by which to increase their profits.

The system was so good that its benefits were expanded to cover more services, such as obstetrics. Companies began to buy policies as fringe benefits for their employees. Everyone was happy with the system.

With the 1960s and the civil rights movement, medical care became a "right." Surely, those who could not afford a private physician or medical insurance deserved access to the "miracles" of modern medicine. The "poor" with the greatest need were the elderly with their limited incomes and multiple medical problems. Thus, Medicare was implemented into the Social Security system.

Again, those involved were happy, and there were few problems. Soon, Medicaid for the non-elderly indigent was added as a federally and state-financed program.

The field of medicine underwent explosive growth. More available money meant expanded facilities and services. This created a shortage of physicians, so medical school classes almost doubled in size. More available money meant increased investments in new diagnostic procedures, drugs and other forms of treatment. The promises of cures prompted the federal government to spend billions of dollars for medical research.

Today, "we the people of the United States" now spend over 12 percent of our Gross National Product on the "nurture" of the human body. (Could this figure in some sense be considered a tithe to what we worship?)

Philosophy and Theology Are Important

Hindsight is better than foresight, so this side of the problem makes an analysis easier. In most quarters, however, the roots of the problem still go unrecognized, because one's anthropology or philosophy of who and what man is determines social and governmental policy.

Many errors were made, but I will limit myself to four that are major. First, and possibly the greatest, was the hope of science. Because such technical sophistication and success had occurred in other fields of science, it was generally assumed that the same progress was possible in medicine. A vision of a physical utopia without pain and disease abounded (and continues today). Mostly subconscious, but sometimes clearly stated, was the hope of immortality.

That vision and hope today are complete failures. For example, the "war on cancer" has not made the first step of progress against any major killer in this category.

The Bible says that God's curse upon mankind is the cause of death (Genesis 2:16-17, 3:19; Hebrews 9:27).[12] It is fascinating to see that graphs of the ages of death of various populations of the past and the present *all* show an upper limit of 80-90 years. This evidence shows that medical care or living conditions have no effect on longevity. Thus, the statistical and Biblical evidence is conclusive that man cannot thwart God's curse.

Second, the relationship between morality (i.e., Biblical ethics) and health has been almost entirely ignored. Payments by both the government and private insurance have virtually no limitations for the consequences of sin (the only exception is higher premiums on smokers). The costs of medical care for immorality are staggering, as sexually transmitted diseases are epidemic, and ectopic pregnancies (caused by these diseases) have quadrupled in the last 30 years. Alcoholism causes rampant disease and death. Tobacco use causes one-third of all cancers. Homicide and suicide are among the top killers. Heart disease is aggravated by obesity, smoking, stress, and a lack of exercise.

Third, the subjective dimension of health removes any restriction on the "need" for medical care. For example, a person may have recurrent or chronic headaches. Most are muscle-contraction (tension) headaches. Yet, no test has yet been or will be developed to determine the degree of pain that a person feels. As long as the headache is there, the person is "eligible" for the maximum diagnostic and therapeutic benefits available through insurance or the government. Other forms of insurance have objective measurements: the ashes of a house (fire insurance), the twisted metal of a car (auto insurance), and the body of a dead person (life insurance). The objective evidence of a headache or a myriad of other aches, pains and disabilities have few, and in some cases, no objective evidence.

Fourth, the role of government in medicine is doubtful, at

least to the degree that it is involved today. One Biblical role of government in medical care seems to be the control of infectious diseases, based upon the Priests' role in the Old Testament to regulate leprosy and other diseases (e.g., Leviticus 13). Likely, its role in medicine should be limited to that one area.

The general function of government is supposed to reward good and punish evil (Romans 13:1-7). Certainly, there is no reference anywhere in the Bible that explicitly gives a medical role to the state. As Christians, we are to be charitable in ways that would include medical care, but charity cannot be a function of the government. By definition, charity is voluntary, whereas collection and administration of taxes by the state is backed by the force of the state. Further, the state can use the "good" of its provided medical care to become increasingly dictatorial.[13]

AIDS in This Economic Crisis

The principles that govern these issues determine what should be proposed to provide for the care of AIDS patients. As AIDS has caused us to re-evaluate the use of blood transfusions (Chapter 12), it should cause us to re-evaluate our medical payment system. The crisis has been created because those who have designed the system failed to consider a Biblical understanding of man and government and the subjective aspect of medical problems.

What sort of changes need to be made in our system? As we follow the order of the previous section, the first change concerns the hope of medical science. The biggest hurdle in our ability to give the proper value to medical care is the delusion that modern medicine is effective. While I cannot lay the foundation for that claim here, I and others have done so elsewhere.[14]

I am *not* saying that modern medicine offers nothing of value. I *am* saying that we need to select carefully what is valuable -- and omit the rest.

I am also saying that modern medicine has greatly contributed to modern diseases and death. For example, since 1973, the medical profession (in general and officially) has championed the cause of the homosexuals as an "alternative lifestyle." All recent medical students and physicians have been vigorously taught that their interaction with patients should be "non-judgmental." That advocacy of medicine helped bring about the current plague. The disease and death that have resulted should be *subtracted* from any gains that are perceived in medicine. The same could be said for the epidemic of other sexually transmitted diseases and abortions.

I am even willing to make the radical statement that *a total collapse of the medical care system in the United States today would not seriously affect the overall health of the population.* In many ways, our health would be improved. Now, I do not hope for that, but I do hope for a reformation within medicine towards Biblical guidelines.

The second needed change is to realize that health is primarily an issue of morality. The same mistake has been made as in public education: that medicine (and education) can be practiced (taught) without a system of morality. It is time to reward the moral person with a payment system designed to reflect his healthy lifestyle and to require the immoral person to pay more heavily for his own care.

The third area is more difficult, but we have to wrestle with stricter limits on payments for subjective symptoms that are consistent with non-physical disease and are without objective evidence of a physical basis.

Fourth, the role of government in personal medical care must be phased out. The government has promoted immorality (and the disease and death that it has caused) right along with the medical profession. Further, it has forcibly (through taxation) caused us to subsidize this immorality. Surely, there are needs to be met by those who cannot afford basic care. This legitimate need, however, does not mean that it is the responsibility of the government to provide it.

Let us remember that the word "hospital" came from "hospice" -- or places of refuge that the Church and other groups of Christians developed and sponsored. Many hospitals (Catholic and Protestant) retain their denominational names. They were once entirely supported by their Church and charities. Now they are supported by the gigantic insurance and government payment systems. In many ways they have capitulated to these third-party payers to remain solvent.

What To Do

AIDS has focused our attention on problems that were already severe, but less obvious. To address these problems only as they relate to AIDS is inadequate. Perhaps, some momentum for reform will be forthcoming because of AIDS. If so, we should move toward a more complete reform of the whole system. Where possible, we should support the private development of insurance plans that place strict limits on life-style. We simply cannot afford to continue to pay for the disease and death that is caused by the wanton pursuit of pleasure.

We should not let the specter of rising medical costs blind us to increasing government control of medical care. The situation is now obvious that government is an enemy of quality medical care. Freedom to practice medicine and free choice of the patient and his physician are being severely limited under federal and state regulations. Sometimes the physician even faces severe financial penalties and criminal prosecution! We must remember the Economic Golden Rule: "He who has the gold makes the rules."

Notes and References

1. Rebecca Voelker, "AIDS Spending to Double by 1994," *American Medical News* 33 (July 20, 1990):3, 36.

2. David E. Bloom and Geoffrey Carliner, "The Economic Impact of AIDS in the United States," *Science* 239 (February 5, 1988):604-610. This article gives a comprehensive overview of all the costs of AIDS.

3. Growth for the past 18 months (as this book is written) has been toward the lower figure, increasing this magnitude of lost productivity.

4. Medicaid is administered jointly by the states and the federal government and provides payment for medical services for low-income individuals and families.

5. No author. *The Augusta [Georgia] Chronicle* (June 18, 1987), 5C.

6. No author. "AIDS Impact Mounting, Insurers Say," *American Medical News* 31 (February 5, 1988), 35.

7. No author. "HIV Test Use Linked to Fall in Claims Paid," *American Medical News* 32 (October 20, 1989):32.

8. Deborah S. Pinkney, "Public Hospitals Bear Brunt of AIDS Care Burden," *American Medical News* 31 (July 1, 1988):2, 8.

9. Susan Adelman, "Will AIDS Be the Death of Inner-City Hospitals?" *American Medical News* 31 (November 11, 1988):29, 32.

10. As an aside, I have difficulty with the idea of a "chance" encounter with HIV. There are several stories of Christians and other "upright" citizens becoming infected with HIV from a "one-night stand" in an otherwise faithful marriage. The chances of this occurrence are on the order of one in a thousand. Although infection from one such contact is possible, the more likely explanation is repetitive adultery.

11. Those back issues are July 1987, October 1987, April 1988, and July 1988. They are available for $4.00 each from JBEM, P.O. Box 13231, Florence, SC 29504-3231.

12. Many conservative theologians believe that Adam and Eve were created to live forever, had they not sinned. Even after the Fall, their descendants lived for hundreds of years. After the Flood, however, this longevity fell off considerably to the 80-90 year range.

13. George Yossif, "Catastrophic Legislation," *The New American* 4 (May 9, 1988):31-38. This article is an excellent analysis of how the government increases its control over people and their resources through medical care. A reprint may be obtained by writing *The New American*, 395 Concord Ave., Belmont, MA 02178.

14. Franklin E. Payne, *Biblical/Medical Ethics*, (Milford, Michigan: Mott Media, 1985), 33-49. I discuss at length the ineffectiveness of medical care. Also, see Leonard S. Sagan, *The Health of Nations: True Causes of Sickness and Well-Being*, (New York: Basic Books, 1987).

CHAPTER 11

What About Quarantine and Universal Testing?

Many conservatives and evangelical Christians have called for the quarantine of HIV-infected people. There is a precedent for such a call. Historically, quarantine has been a standard of public health policy for centuries. Quarantine signs could be seen on houses as late as the 1950s, as many readers will recall. Quarantine, however, has been rejected by "officials" as a means to control the AIDS epidemic.

Two questions, then, need to be addressed. First, can quarantine be defended as a Biblical position? Second, is quarantine applicable to the AIDS epidemic, in spite of official opposition?

A Biblical Perspective on Quarantine

> "As for the leper who has the infection, his clothes shall be torn, and the hair of his head shall be uncovered, and he shall cover his mustache and cry, 'Unclean! Unclean!' He shall remain unclean all the days during which he has the infection; he is unclean. He shall live alone; his dwelling shall be outside the camp" (Leviticus 13:45-46, NASB).

Chapters 13 and 14 of Leviticus are devoted in their entirety to public health policies, administered by the Priests. Clearly, these are principles of public health, giving Priests the power to quarantine people (13:4-5, 50) and to destroy property (even houses) to control the spread of a dreaded disease (13:52, 14:45). In fact, the argument has been made that "The laws against leprosy may be regarded as the first model of sanitary legislation."[1] A thorough discussion of such texts and their meaning for modern medicine, however, has not been published (to my knowledge).

This text presents some difficulties in its interpretation. First, it contains ceremonial practices along with the public health measures. These practices do not have any medicinal value, as they have no physical application to the infected person himself (Leviticus 14:4-7, 10-32, 49-53). Thus, some discernment is needed to determine which passages may be applied as public health measures and which should not. Almost all Christians agree that the ceremonial practices of the Mosaic Law were abrogated with the perfect sacrifice of Jesus Christ.

Second, the leprosy described in both the Old and New Testaments is not the disease that we call by the same name today.[2] Modern leprosy is not highly contagious, where Biblical leprosy *was* highly contagious, (at least it was thought to be). Likely, Biblical leprosy was one of several skin diseases to which the general term "leprosy" was applied.

Third, the state of Israel was a theocracy. That is, it was governed directly by God through the Levites, judges, kings and prophets. Obviously, the United States is not a theocracy. Thus, the Priests' role in leprosy could not exactly correspond to that of the public health officer of today.

Despite these difficulties (and others), we can at least establish from the Bible that the government has some role in the control of infectious diseases, including quarantine. This conclusion seems consistent with the interpretation of Leviticus 13-14 and other texts in the Old Testament Law by many Christians presently and historically.

Quarantine and HIV/AIDS

Some diseases are more contagious than others, so there is no reason to quarantine (or to place in isolation, as it is more commonly called today) those diseases that are not readily transmitted from one person to another. As we have seen, HIV is highly infectious only to those who are sexually immoral and abuse IV-drugs.[3] Outside of these groups, HIV is not highly infectious, that is, it is not casually transmitted (except possibly in rare and unusual situations). Thus, there seems to be no reason to quarantine HIV-infected patients for fear of HIV transmission.

Quarantine is also impossible without universal testing, because quarantine requires that those people infected with HIV be found. Universal testing has considerable hurdles to overcome. (See later section.)

Health-Care Workers and Other Patients

What may not be understood is that a kind of quarantine is already being applied to AIDS patients. *Any measure of infection control is a form of quarantine.* These measures are commonly applied in hospitals, nursing homes, and other institutions. While the number of health-care workers who have become infected with HIV is small (relatively) and no patients have been documented to have acquired HIV from other patients (see Chapter 9), AIDS patients *are* reservoirs of infections other than HIV. Since most patients with AIDS are homosexuals and IV-drug abusers, they are also infected with hepatitis B, intestinal parasites, and a variety of other sexually transmitted diseases. Also, there is an increasing number of AIDS patients with tuberculosis.

As the number of HIV-infected patients increases, the number of health-care workers infected with HIV from patients will also increase. Many nurses and others will quit their jobs (many already have) where they are continually exposed to AIDS patients. If more reasonable measures that protect health-care workers are not instituted, a real crisis in manpower may occur in health-care institutions. A shortage of health-care workers already exists, and a further decrease will aggravate the available care for non-AIDS patients.

Further, the presence of health-care workers *who are HIV positive because of risk behaviors* is a potential source of infection to patients.[4] Almost 6 percent of people with AIDS are health-care workers. This percent almost exactly corresponds to the percentage of health-care workers in the U.S. population. Thus, some 4800 (over 60 percent have died) of these are presently caring for patients. If the same 6 percent applies to HIV-infected people who have not yet progressed to AIDS, then approximately 60,000 HIV-positive health-care workers are now caring for non-HIV-infected patients.

The situation is one of an increasing concentration of people with AIDS in hospitals and other institutions. It is here that infection control needs to be applied.

How to do it? Separate hospital wards and/or separate facilities are possibilities. I do not have space here to discuss in detail how these separate facilities might be developed, but likely something on the order of a hospice will be necessary because of cost and the rapid deployment that is needed. Home care should also be developed.[5]

Again, such plans seem sorely lacking among medical care planners. Even in New York City, where the crisis is perhaps the worst anywhere, leaders are mostly scratching their heads instead of taking action.

It would also seem appropriate for those who are infected because of their immorality to bear more of the burden of this epidemic, and thus demonstrate the "love" which homosexuals say that they possess. Those who are HIV-positive, but without symptoms, could participate in the care of those who have AIDS to avoid unnecessary exposure of the uninfected. At the Medical College of Georgia, such a plan is being explored for a dental student who has been found to be HIV-positive.

Precautions for Children in Day-Care Centers

While studies show the safety of "casual exposures" within households to HIV-infected people (Chapter 9), there seems to be no reason to take unnecessary risks in day-care centers. Small children often have open sores, they drool, they urinate and defecate unexpectedly and sometimes profusely, and in other ways are contaminated with their own and others' "body fluids."

Further, a 12-month study of children (ages 0-6 years) in day-care centers showed that 104 of a total of 224 children were bitten at least once (some more than once), with a total of 347 bites.[6] While the study did not measure the severity of the bites, the potential for the transmission of HIV and other diseases is real, even though it may be remote. In a nursery environment where children are limited to their own cribs, I see no danger of one child's infecting another when routine hygienic measures are followed by adult workers.

Incorrigible HIV Carriers

One of the few areas that conservatives and liberals can agree upon is the prosecution of HIV carriers who know that they are positive and yet attempt to donate blood or continue to have sexual relationships without telling their partners that they are HIV-positive. Twenty states have enacted statutes permitting the prosecution of persons whose behavior poses a risk of HIV transmission, first recommended by the President's Commission on AIDS under President Ronald Reagen.[7]

> "In the vast majority of instances, such prosecutions have resulted either in acquittal or in a decision to drop the case. When there have been guilty verdicts, the penalties have at times been unusually harsh."[8]

The Major Issue: Homosexuality and IV-Drug Abuse

The major issue concerning infection control is the morality and legality of homosexuality and IV-drug abuse, as well as a return to sexual morality and the traditional family as the basic unit of society. You can imagine trying to restrict the lifestyle of a homosexual in today's political climate. Officials recoil from the possible violation of the confidentiality of a positive HIV test. They would not even entertain the idea of overt identification for control of someone with a positive test.

The key, then, to the quarantine of any patients with AIDS is the defeat of the protectionism of the homosexuals. This defeat is key not only to the AIDS crisis, but also to the future morality and health of our country. Christians must face the question of the freedom of homosexuals vs. restriction of their activities. To allow them their current degree of freedom is to allow them to influence and recruit other boys and men into their lifestyle and continue to spread their diseases. (See Chapter 5.)

Other Obstacles to Quarantine

Even if a general quarantine of people with HIV/AIDS were necessary because of the infectious pattern of HIV, our culture has so slipped in its moral moorings that implementation of the quarantine without other major social changes would not be possible. Some examples of these obstacles are the following.

1) The practice of medicine is morally corrupt. Abortion is defended by the AMA, the largest organization of physicians. Homosexuality is endorsed by the American Psychiatric Association. Condoms are preached, instead of sexual abstinence.

2) Our whole culture is sexually promiscuous. Who is willing to condemn others, if they are guilty themselves?

3) We have been unable to control or treat IV-drug abuse. What is there to offer any glimmer of hope that we may be able to do so in the future?

4) We have a health-care system that requires no moral responsibility of its participants. The person with cancer of the breast (a disease unrelated to moral acts) receives the same insurance and government benefits and payments as the person with cirrhosis of the liver (a disease commonly related to alcoholism).

5) The loss of freedom that would come with quarantine for everyone would likely wreak a far greater cost to the "innocents" of this epidemic than what we are now experiencing. (See "Let's Be Careful..." below.)

For now, quarantine is not an issue for conservatives. There are many more pertinent and protective areas to influence. We must continue to agitate for the same application of public health measures to AIDS as to other infectious and sexually transmitted diseases and cry out against the presence of open homosexuality in our society.

AIDS is a symptom of the moral disease of our society. We must work to restore those Biblical values that honor God and which made our nation strong and healthy. Physical health, like economic health, cannot come about by government action, primarily, but by personal moral responsibility.

Universal Testing

Universal testing involves the testing of every man, woman, and child in the United States. Many conservatives have called for such testing as a public health measure to limit the spread of the AIDS epidemic.

The Tests

Two tests are being widely used to screen for HIV. New tests that are more specific and more sensitive have been developed, but it is not yet clear which (if any) would replace these two primary tests for mass screening. What *is* clear is that the new tests are considerably more expensive, thus increasing the costs for any major screening program.[9]

The first test used to check for the presence of HIV is the ELISA (enzyme linked immunosorbent assay), sometimes abbreviated EIA (enzyme immunoassay). The second test (used to confirm the EIA) is the WB (Western Blot). Both test for the presence of *antibody* to HIV, not the virus itself. That is, when HIV infects the body, certain cells identify the viral proteins as foreign substances and produce antibodies against them.[10] It is these antibodies that the tests detect, not the virus itself.

The period of time ("window") when the virus is present *without* the presence of antibodies is one major limitation of these tests. A person can be *infected* and *infectious*, but these two tests will not be positive until the immune system manufactures antibodies. It is for this reason that the blood supply still is not entirely safe from HIV (Chapter 12). Further, this "window" may be present for as long as 3 years in some people.[11]

When one sees a physician and tests are ordered, the whole

process seems simple and straightforward. That is, the test reveals the presence or absence of the disease, and the physician can make decisions based upon that information. Testing, however, is quite the opposite. A test may be a false positive (the test is positive but no disease is actually present) or a false negative (the disease is present but the test failed to detect it).

The *sensitivity* of a test is the probability that the test will be positive in a patient in whom the factor (as a sign of disease) that is tested for is present. This measure determines the rate of false negatives (the disease is present, but the test is negative). If a test is 99 percent sensitive, then in 100 tests on patients *with the disease*, 99 will be (true) positives, and one will be a false negative.

The *specificity* of a test is the probability that the test will be negative in the absence of the disease. This measure determines the rate of false positives (the test is positive where the disease is not present). If a test is 99 percent specific, then of 100 tests on patients *without the disease*, 99 will be (true) negatives, and one will be a false positive.

More False Positives Than True Positives Can Occur

A 99 percent specificity and sensitivity are excellent values for a test. Most medical tests are not nearly as accurate. Still, with this level of accuracy, problems exist when large populations with a low prevalence of disease are tested. For example, in a population where the prevalence of a factor being tested for is 1/10,000 and the test is 99 percent specific, the 1 percent false positives result in 100 false positives (of 10,000 screened), when only one true positive exists.

Where the disease has a prevalence of 1 in 10, tests of the same reliability (in 10,000 tested) would result in 990 true positives and 90 false positives. The contrast of these examples demonstrates the greater usefulness of tests in a population that has a high prevalence of disease.

With such information, calculations on HIV and false positives relative to HIV and marriage testing can be performed.[12] Assumptions for these calculations are: 4 million people get married each year; a 0.1 percent prevalence of HIV infection in this group; and tests that are 99.6 percent specific and sensitive.

* Of the 4,000 people who are infected, 3,984 would be detected.

* Of the expected 3,996,000 who are not infected with HIV, 3,980,016 would actually test negative.

* The testing would miss 16 people who are infected.

* False positive results would be obtained on 15,984 people who are not infected with HIV.

The use of *two* tests increases the chances of a *true* positive. The sequential use of the EIA and WB has achieved false positive rates of 1/100,000.[13] If the entire U.S. population (approximately 250 million) were screened in this manner, then false positives could be limited to 2500 people.

I have focused on the false positives. Obviously, the false negatives would provide problems of their own, primarily in their causing infection where the source would be difficult to trace. I have not gone into variability of interpretation, purity of chemicals used in tests, lack of standardization of procedures, adherence to these standards, and other problems that interfere with reliable results.

My estimate is that false positives would actually number 25,000 to 50,000 (from a screen of the entire U.S. population) and a similar number of equivocal tests. These people with false positives would not know that they actually were not infected with HIV for as long as 20 years. Thus, they would live under the fear of AIDS until enough time had passed or new tests were developed to confirm their not being infected.

The occurrence of false positives and other problems with methods of testing are *alone* insufficient to prevent universal testing, *if it were clearly indicated for other reasons*. Before I come to any conclusion, however, I want to explore other relevant issues.

More Arguments Against Universal Testing

A call for universal testing is markedly deficient without reasons that would promote personal or public health. Otherwise, we know who is infected and who is not, but nothing would change concerning the pattern of the spread of HIV. There are at least three such reasons that someone could propose, but I argue against them. First, the forced quarantine of everyone who tests positive. My opposition to this plan except in certain situations has already been stated (above).

Second, we would know precisely how many people are infected. It is doubtful, however, that universal testing will reveal much that we do not already know of the various populations that have been tested.

Third, non-infected individuals would be able to identify those who might infect them. Health-care workers could be more conscientious to follow "universal precautions." Sex partners could have some assurance that the other was HIV-negative. I believe, however, that these people should take upon themselves responsibility for screening their sex partners without imposing such screens for those who are innocent of such immorality.

How Should HIV-Positives Be Identified?

A real problem, however, is how to identify those who are positive and those who are not. Papers or cards could be issued, but these are easily forged, lost, or stolen. In emergencies, such identification may not be readily available.

If we should go to universal testing, tattoos seem the only readily available and reliable method of identification. It is always with the person and any change of it is easily detectable. Where can the tattoo be put? One suggestion has been the inside of the lower lip, normally concealed but easily checked. Too easily, I think. I suggest the top of the shoulder, where it would easily be covered by clothing, but the clothing could be pushed aside discreetly when necessary.

My goal here is not to advocate tattooing[14] (see below), but to point out that those who advocate universal testing must have a reliable and quick way to identify those who test positive. Otherwise, what is the point of testing?

Let's Be Careful -- of Big Brother

Universal testing would necessarily grant extensive powers to the government. First, a system would have to be designed to be sure that everyone was screened. Finding those with permanent addresses is easy enough, but large numbers of those most likely to have HIV (inner-city dwellers, IV-drug abusers, immigrants, prostitutes, etc.) are quite mobile. A comprehensive roundup of all these transients would require considerable social and police efforts. This effort would have to recur in cycles, because infections may occur after the first test or in those who are false negatives.

Government officials have already invaded our homes with their propaganda brochure "Understanding AIDS." With universal testing they would have the power to invade our homes physically. *Universal testing means mandatory testing backed by the full power and authority of the government.* We already know too well that our own government is not only inefficient in the exercise of such power, but often abuses such power. Are we ready to grant it that power now? Are we ready to grant it that power as a precedent to be applied to other problems?

I have not seen this concern addressed by anyone who advocates universal testing. As I have meditated on it, I wonder if the "cure" may be worse than the disease (pun intended), especially because we have considerable evidence that the virus is not transmitted casually.

Another question is whether or not screening *is* the responsibility of the government -- or of families and individuals. I do not have the space here to defend my belief on a Biblical basis, but the Bible seems to place the responsibility for health and protection primarily within the family, and secondarily on the government (Leviticus 13-14). For example, is it unreasonable to expect two people who are engaged to marry to require tests of each other rather than the government's doing so? Christians also need to think seriously about this role of

Big Brother. Perhaps churches should play a role in public health measures as well.[15]

Notes and References

1. Arturo Castiglione, *A History of Medicine*, (New York: Alfred A. Knopf, Inc., 1941):71. Cited in S. I. McMillen and David E. Stern, *None of These Diseases*, (Old Tappan, New Jersey: Fleming H. Revell Company, 1984), 22.

2. Rebecca A. Baillie and E. Eugene Baillie, *Southern Medical Journal* 75 (July 1982):855-857.

3. HIV is also highly infectious to those who receive HIV-infected blood and from an HIV-infected mother to her unborn child, but quarantine is hardly applicable to these situations.

4. I made this statement in the June 1988 issue of my AIDS newsletter. In July 1990, the CDC announced that a Florida dentist had infected one of his patients (and later, 2 more were reported). See Chapter 9.

5. The ineptitude of bureaucracies to handle a real emergency is evident here. I first wrote on this subject 3 years ago, but few effective measures to handle the large increase of AIDS patients have been enacted and implemented. I suspect that the role of churches and other charitable institutions has been considerable in caring for AIDS patients, while city, state, and federal bureaucracies have only muddled along *in spite of massive AIDS funding*.

6. Judith Garrard, *et al.*, "Epidemiology of Human Bites to Children in a Day-Care Center," *American Journal of Diseases in Children* 142 (June 1988):643-650.

7. Ronald Bayer, "Public Health Policy and the AIDS Epidemic: An End to HIV Exceptionalism," *The New England Journal of Medicine* 324 (May 23, 1991):1400-1404.

8. *Ibid.*

9. J. Sanford Schwartz, *et al.*, "Human Immunodeficiency Virus Test Evaluation, Performance, and Use," *The Journal of the American Medical Association* 259 (May 6, 1988):2574-2579. This article thoroughly discusses the various tests for HIV available at that time.

10. See Note 4, p. 105, for more information on the role of antibodies.

11. Laurie Abraham, "Longer Latency Period Poses Questions About HIV Tests," *American Medical News* 31 (June 24, 1988):42-43.

12. Dale Murphy, "AIDS: Pray for Reason," *Consultant* 27 (October 1987):3, 16.

13. H. F. Polesky, "Update: Serologic Testing for Antibody to Human Immunodeficiency Virus," *Morbidity and Mortality Weekly Report* 36 (January 8, 1988):833-840.

14. Tattooing is also proscribed by Scripture (Leviticus 19:28).

15. I must apologize for brevity here. This paragraph is "loaded" with principles, some of which I have discussed previously. I must, however, stop somewhere.

CHAPTER 12

How Safe Is Our Blood Supply?

The most important and the most tragic event concerning the safety of our blood supply was the failure of government and blood bank "officials" to protect the public from HIV-infected blood. That fiasco has already been noted (Chapter 2), but should also be mentioned here.

All the "fallout" from AIDS, however, is not negative. In some areas the threat of AIDS has served to educate people about risks that were already present, but too little was being done about them. A significant area where this positive effect has occurred is the transfusion of blood. *The far greater risk from transfusions is not from HIV but from hepatitis and other complications.* "Not until the AIDS crisis focused attention on the blood supply did the risk of hepatitis come to full public view."[1] Thus, AIDS has caused both physicians and their patients to reconsider the use of blood products in most situations. This re-evaluation has been long overdue. Thus, my focus will be on a whole spectrum of problems with blood transfusions, and not just HIV.

Of Hepatitis and Other Diseases[2]

The most serious complications following blood transfusions are three types of hepatitis, each caused by a different virus: hepatitis A, B, and non-A, non-B (NANB). During the early 1960s, some 33 percent of transfusion recipients became infected with one of these forms of hepatitis. During the 1970s, with the introduction of screening tests for hepatitis B, the incidence was reduced to 15 percent. In mid-1986, indirect testing for NANB was started. Estimates are that, with even newer screens, the risk of hepatitis has been reduced to 1-2 percent.[3] Hepatitis, however, remains the most common of the serious problems that can occur with transfusions.

Hepatitis A is rare in blood transfusions because it is an acute illness that has no chronic carriers. Hepatitis B comprises 10-20 percent of transfusion-acquired hepatitis, in spite of tests to screen out this disease. NANB comprises 80-90 percent of transfusion hepatitis.[4] In 50 percent of NANB cases, chronic hepatitis will develop, and 10 percent will acquire cirrhosis of the liver (severe destruction of the liver that is eventually fatal).

Other serious transfusion complications include circulatory overload in patients with heart disease, acute lung injury (a direct effect on the lung itself), hemolysis (the destruction of red blood cells [RBCs]), accumulation of iron, and malaria and other infections (not already named). Individually, these complications occur in less than 1 in 10,000 transfusions. The chance of any one during a given transfusion would be 1 in 1000.

Adverse effects that are not serious, but "troublesome" (i.e., may range from temporarily debilitating to asymptomatic, but almost never cause a serious or chronic illness), include a reduction of the RBC production in the bone marrow, positive blood tests for some diseases that the patient has never had (i.e., false positives, see Chapter 11), production of various antibodies, fevers, chills, allergic reactions and delayed hemolysis. As to frequency of these problems, a decrease in the production of RBCs occurs "frequently," new antibody production may occur in 10 percent of transfusions, and the other problems occur in less than one percent of transfusions. Taken together, however, one or more of these complications will appear in 20 percent of transfusions.

In addition to blood typing, crossmatching, and tests for hepatitis, all donated blood is screened for syphilis, cytomegalovirus and HIV. Because of positive tests with these screens, 12 percent of all units (one unit is approximately one pint) are discarded and the donor notified of the positive test results.

HIV and the Blood Supply

With the above background, we can now turn to the subject of HIV and blood transfusions. Keep in mind that we are discussing the transmission of HIV via blood products and not AIDS *per se*, which occurs several years after the initial infection with HIV. (See Chapter 3.)

The ELISA and Western Blot, two tests for antibodies to HIV, were instituted on all donated blood in March 1985. (See page 26.) Many argued for indirect tests prior to the availability of the ELISA and the Western Blot, but the protests of the blood banks and the homosexual lobbies prevented their introduction. Thus, many thousands of HIV infections could have been prevented. The number of persons infected with HIV via blood transfusions (computations here will include hemophiliacs, although the CDC lists them in a separate category) has been estimated to be as high as 30,000, with 7200 in 1984 alone.

Through January 31, 1991, however, *a total of 5543 adults and children had been diagnosed with AIDS which had been acquired through blood transfusions*. This number is not likely to rise much higher for the reason that infection with HIV via blood products is now rare. *Almost all those who were infected prior to antibody testing for HIV have already died* (see below).

(When I first wrote on this subject in August 1988, I predicted that this total would "peak within the next 2-3 years and then begin to decline." At that time, there were 2585 people infected from blood transfusions; there have been 1406 more since that time. While my prediction was accurate, the tragedy is that many of these were needlessly infected.)

That's the background, but what is the threat of infection with HIV in the blood supply today? All blood is screened by the ELISA test. "Positives" are then screened with the Western Blot. These tests, however, may have false negatives, that is, the virus may be present, but the test is negative. This negative result may occur for two reasons. 1) An error may occur in the test itself or in the testing procedure. 2) HIV can be present before antibodies are produced ("window" of infectivity). Usually, this period of time is 6-14 weeks, but it has been reported to be as long as 3 1/2 years. In addition, 4 men with AIDS have been found to have converted their antibody tests from *positive to negative*, while more direct tests show that HIV is present.[5]

The number of these false negatives is quite small. With a rate of positives among all blood donors of 1/10,000 (actually it is less), and a false negative rate of 1/100 (actually the tests are better than this), then in 1 million donors there would be only one false negative because of the test itself. Worst-case estimates place the rate at 4-5 per million.

One researcher has placed the number who pass through the "window" period at 26 per million units of blood collected, or 1 in 38,000 units.[6] With 18 million blood components transfused each year, there is the possibility of approximately 470 people annually who could become infected with HIV via blood transfusions. Only 4 million patients actually receive transfusions each year, and each patient who is transfused receives an average of 3-5 units. These multiple transfusions increase the possibility of infection to 1/12,000 to 1/8,000 *per transfusion*.

An actual study shows a similar incidence. The actual rate of seroconversion (from HIV-negative to HIV-positive) was calculated over a 2-year period in Los Angeles and Orange Counties, California. Researchers calculated that "the risk of HIV transmission from an HIV-seronegative unit was 1 in 102,000 to 1 in 51,000 (with a best guess of 1/68,000)."[7] The incidence of 1/38,000 and 1/68,000 are really closer than they seem when one considers the extrapolations and assumptions that must be assumed to arrive at these numbers.

Many patients who become infected with HIV via blood transfusions do not live long enough to progress to AIDS. In one study, 40 percent of patients who received HIV-infected blood died from the condition (e.g., a bleeding intestinal ulcer) that caused the need for their transfusion, before any effect of HIV manifested itself.[8] This statistic should not detract from concern about HIV transmission, but it does show that the conditions that require transfusions are often life-threatening in themselves.

Will You Ever Need Blood?

The chances are good that each of us will need a transfusion at some time in our lives. For example, there are approximately 250 million people in the United States, with 3-4 million people getting blood products each year. If everyone transfused each year had not been transfused before, in 70 years, every American would have had a transfusion. Of course, many diseases require multiple transfusions over a long period of time, so this projection is inaccurate. It would seem plausible, however, that any one person stands a 30-50 percent chance of needing a blood transfusion in his or her lifetime.

How to Avoid Transfusion Risks

1) *Don't have a transfusion!* I am neither being sarcastic nor taking the position of some cults that blood transfusions are wrong. The truth is that many transfusions are not necessary. Perhaps, the association of blood as a necessity for life prompts physicians to overlook the risks, while patients (and their families) are comforted from the dramatic appearance of blood being infused.

In one study, 1930 units of blood or blood products were used in 560 patients, involving 765 episodes of transfusions.[9] "By clearly defined, present criteria, 42.3 percent of the episodes were found not to be appropriate." Patients most prone to inappropriate use were those with end-stage kidney disease, terminal cancer, and cancer patients on chemotherapy. "Most unjustified episodes occurred as a result of the overestimation of the immediate risk incurred by withholding transfusion."

Physicians need to consider seriously *not* giving blood every time they think about using it. For elective surgery and other non-emergency situations, patients should ask their physicians whether a transfusion is really necessary, if such is mentioned as a possibility. (You might also want to discuss whether the surgery is really necessary in the first place *and* get a second opinion!)

I do not want to diminish the life-saving nature of blood transfusions, or the fact that in many instances they cannot be avoided. Physicians, however, can eliminate some instances where blood transfusions are not really necessary and reduce these risks to their patients.

2) *Store your own blood.* Such storage can be short-term or long-term. If elective (non-emergency) surgery requires the presence of blood for possible transfusion, the surgery may be scheduled to allow enough time to store 2-3 units of your own blood to be given, if necessary, during or after the surgery. This practice is called *autologous transfusion*. Since stored blood must be used within 5 weeks of the time that it is donated (if it is not frozen), there are time restrictions on this method. The frequency that such blood can be used is increasing all the time, as physicians continue to test the surgical procedures for which autologous blood can be used. (See the following.)

Blood can be frozen for 10 years or longer. (Exactly how long is not yet known, because this technology has not been available long enough for its time limit to be determined.) Some commercial firms will store frozen blood for you and your family in case of a future need. The advantages are obvious.

The disadvantages are considerable. a) The cost is likely to be greater than $150 per unit per year. Since the average transfusion is 3-5 units, storing only one unit is virtually useless. b) An emergency is an emergency. Your blood would have to be moved from storage, thawed, and transported to your geographic location.

I do not recommend this route for those who do not already have some medical problem for which a blood transfusion is very likely at some time in the future.[10]

3) *Have your physicians give you back your blood lost during surgery -- another form of autologous transfusion.*[11] "Perioperative blood salvage" is performed during an operation by washing the blood out of sponges, saving that which is obtained from suction, etc. Then it is filtered and given back to the patient during the surgery itself or at a later time, if needed.

4) *Have your physicians dilute your blood, also a method of autologous transfusion.* "Acute normovolemic hemodilu-

tion" is the withdrawal of blood immediately prior to surgery so that any blood lost during surgery contains fewer red blood cells per unit. Then after surgery, the withdrawn blood is transfused back.

The application of such measures was studied in the Department of Surgery at Michael Reese Hospital and Medical Center in Chicago, where 161 patients had orthopedic (80 percent) or vascular (20 percent) surgery under their autologous blood program.[12] Preoperative and perioperative blood salvage methods (described above) were used with an average yield of 4.3 units of blood for each patient. Of these patients, 61 needed additional blood, but their physicians believe that additional measures will eliminate almost 60 percent of those in the future.[13]

These procedures are not without inherent risks, but they are considerably less risky than transfusions of someone else's blood.

5) *Do not select your own donors.* At first glance, donations from friends and relatives seems to be a good potential source for blood, especially in emergencies. The underlying assumption is that this blood carries less risk of infection to the recipient. In reality, this blood is not likely to be better than that from the general donor population -- and it may be worse!

In a study of almost 500,000 donated units, the risk that a blood donation from a first-time "directed" donor will be positive for hepatitis B is 2.8 times the risk from a volunteer unit.[14] This risk for units from "directed" donors who had previously donated, however, was less than the volunteer units. (The statistical validity of this comparison was uncertain.)

The authors offer this possible explanation. All first-time donors have a higher prevalence of transmissible diseases. If they find that they test positive for a screened disease, then they will be unlikely to donate again. However, they might donate again under the covert or overt pressure to donate for a person that they know or love, to avoid having to admit that they have a transmissible disease. My recommendation is *when a transfusion cannot be avoided and an autologous method is not possible*, that blood be accepted from what is available at your hospital.

The only benefit from directed donations is that the number of donated units can be credited to a designated patient, thereby reducing his medical costs.

Good News and Bad News

The bad news is that the AIDS epidemic has caused a slight decline in blood donations.[15] This decline represents a reversal of a 30-year trend upward. The good news is that transfusions of whole blood and platelets *decreased* almost 3-fold from 1982-1986. Rates for plasma transfusions decreased 4-fold. One expert stated, "Physicians were thinking more about the risks to their patients of a transfusion.... These changes have their primary roots in the dynamics of the AIDS epidemic...."[16]

Also, the increase in autologous transfusions was "phenomenal," increasing almost 10-fold from 1982-1986. "Potentially, up to 50 percent of patients (in non-emergency situations) can use autologous donations."[17] AIDS, then, seems to have caused changes in transfusion practices that other diseases have not been able to effect. These two changes represent positive effects of what is mostly a severely tragic epidemic.

In Conclusion

There are definite risks associated with blood transfusions. HIV may be the worst, but it is one of the least likely. NANB hepatitis and hepatitis B are by far the most common, serious and possibly fatal diseases to be acquired in this way.

Christians without known disease or risks, then, should regularly donate their blood to increase the pool of "good" blood. Some donors fear the possibility of a false positive test for HIV, but the chance of this error is quite minimal. (See Chapter 11.) The fear that one can acquire HIV from donating is also unrealistic.[18]

AIDS has caused many physicians and lay people to be more cautious with blood transfusions and to implement better and safer procedures. This improvement, however, has been at the cost of the thousands who acquired HIV *before* blood screening began. There are few "silver linings" to the dark cloud of AIDS and homosexual advocacy, but changes in transfusion practices represent one of these bright spots.

Practical Steps

1. If you are healthy and have none of the diseases that disqualify you as a donor, give regularly. Make an appointment with a hospital or blood bank and make a note on your personal calendar. The more healthy and morally pure people that donate, the safer our blood supply will be.

2. Learn more about autologous transfusions. Write: Coordinator, NBREP, National Heart, Lung, and Blood Institute, Bldg. 31, Room 3A05, Bethesda, MD 20892 and ask for a reprint of "The Use of Autologous Blood." There is no cost.

Notes and References

1. John Pekkanen, "How Safe Is Our Blood Supply?," *Reader's Digest*, 133 (July 1988):37-44.

2. Richard H. Walker, "Special Report: Transfusion Risks," *American Journal of Clinical Pathology*, 88 (September 1987):374-378. This article gives an excellent summary of the problems of blood transfusions and served as the primary source for the information that I have presented here.

3. Marsha F. Goldsmith, "Blood Bank Officials Hope Altruism Will Pass New (Anti-HCV) Test," *The Journal of the American Medical Association*, 263 (April 4, 1990):1749-1750.

4. *Ibid.* A single agent, named "hepatitis C," has now been identified and likely comprises 90 percent of these post-transfusion cases of hepatitis.

5. Homayoon Farzadegan, "Loss of Human Immunodeficiency Virus Type 1 (HIV-1) Antibodies With Evidence of Viral Infection in Asymptomatic Homosexual Men," *Annals of Internal Medicine* 108 (June 1988):785-790.

6. John W. Ward, "Transmission of Human Immunodeficiency Virus (HIV) by Blood Transfusions Screened as Negative for HIV Antibody," *The New England Journal of Medicine*, 318 (February 25, 1988):473-478.

7. Steven Kleinman *et al.*, "Risk of Human Immunodeficiency Virus Transmission by Anti-HIV Negative Blood: Estimates Using the Lookback Methodology," *Transfusion*, 28 (September-October, 1988):499-501.

8. Herbert A. Perkins, "Risk of AIDS for Recipients of Blood Components From Donors Who Subsequently Developed AIDS," *Blood*, 70 (November 1987):1604-1610.

9. B. Mozes, *et al.*, "Evaluation of the Appropriateness of Blood and Blood Product Transfusion Using Preset Criteria," *Transfusion*, 29 (July-August 1989):473-476.

10. For more information, write Personal Blood Storage, 2427 Forsythe Road, Orlando, FL 32807. I know nothing about this company except that they have subscribed to my AIDS newsletter. They can, however, be a resource for those who are interested in this area.

11. National Blood Resource Program, "The Use of Autologous Blood," *The Journal of the American Medical Association*, 263 (January 19, 1990):414-417.

12. Marsha F. Goldsmith, "As More Surgeons Opt for Autologous Transfusion Route, What's Ahead?," *The Journal of the American Medical Association*, 262 (December 8, 1989):3101-3102.

13. The use of recombinant erythropoietin, a synthetic replica of the hormone that stimulates the bone marrow to make red blood cells, is being studied. When this hormone is given before surgery, the body will begin to produce more RBCs than normal, thus increasing the number available to be salvaged during surgery.

14. Jane M. Starkey, *et al.*, "Markers for Transfusion-Transmitted Disease in Different Groups of Blood Donors," *The Journal of the American Medical Association*, 262 (December 22/29, 1989):3452-3454.

15. Charles Marwick, "Six-Year Slowing Noted in Previously Growing Rate of U.S. Blood Collections," *The Journal of the American Medical Association*, 261 (February 17, 1989):968-969; Janice Somerville, "HIV Prevalence Spurs Boom in Autologous Donations," *American Medical News*, 32 (February 17, 1989):12; Douglas MacN. Surgenor, *et al.*, "Collection and Transfusion of Blood in the United States," *The New England Journal of Medicine*, 322 (June 7, 1990):1646-1651.

16. Marwick, "Six-Year Slowing...," 969.

17. Somerville, "HIV Prevalence Spurs...," 12.

18. The only possibility by which a person could be infected with HIV while giving blood is via the spring-loaded lancet that blood bank personnel use to stick the donor's finger. The lancet is disposable; the spring-loaded holder is not. While no case of HIV transmission has been reported via this route, cases of hepatitis B have been. The source was blood on the device itself, not the lancet. All that is required for donor safety is for the donor to actually see the technician clean the upper and lower portions of the device at the end where the lancet is contained.

CHAPTER 13

An AIDS Vaccine: Technical and Moral Problems

One major hope for the AIDS epidemic is a vaccine that will be safe and effective. It has been widely broadcast that such a vaccine is not likely to be available before the end of this century, if ever. Thus, we will explore some reasons for the difficulties involved in its development and deployment. Further, we will consider the moral principles that bear on this issue, a subject rarely discussed relative to an HIV vaccine.

Technical Problems

When a "germ"[1] infects a person, the body's immune system identifies this organism as a protein that is foreign to itself. Thus, it develops anti-proteins or *antibodies* that bind with the foreign protein that has been identified. This binding will kill the invading organism or neutralize it so that other body defenses can overcome it.

This process, however, may take days or weeks. Over that time, the person may experience nothing, mild signs and symptoms, or a severe illness. Once the antibodies are formed, the specialized cells of the body that are responsible "remember" the foreign protein, so that in the future they can mount a more rapid defense against that organism. This is the way that immunity develops to such childhood diseases as chicken pox, measles, and mumps.

Vaccines stimulate the body's immune system to develop antibodies against a particular infectious agent, so that the "program" for the antibodies is already present when the organism invades. Thus, the organism is rapidly neutralized and killed before it can cause any illness.

The development of antibodies and vaccines is much more complex than I have described it here, however. While we cannot review all possible approaches, we can cover the ones that are most likely to be used to develop a vaccine against HIV.

There are eight different products that can be used to stimulate antibodies against HIV: live attenuated HIV, whole inactivated HIV, live recombinant viruses, synthetic viruses, natural products, recombinant DNA products, anti-idiotypes, and passive immunization. It is beyond the scope of this book to go into each of these, but my cited reference goes into necessary detail for those interested.[2]

Researchers must choose which one of these eight products they will research, then choose the particular variety of each, and finally the technique of administration. Thus, the number of possible approaches is almost endless. Each researcher will choose according to such factors as his own experience, the experience of others in his field, and the available money for a particular approach.

Once the product and technique are determined and the vaccine is produced, it must meet a series of requirements from the Food and Drug Administration (FDA) relative to purity, composition, and stability. Further, research in animals must show that the vaccine is safe and immunogenic (produces the requisite antibodies).

Considerable debate in the scientific community has centered around whether protective immunity must be shown in an animal model system before beginning studies in humans. That is, the vaccine must not only stimulate antibody production, it must do so sufficiently to prevent actual infection with HIV and meet certain standards of safety. Currently, researchers are not fulfilling this step because: 1) a standard by which to evaluate protective immunity is lacking, 2) HIV does not affect any experimental animal exactly as it does a human, 3) the spreading pandemic demands urgency, and 4) additional clinical information about the immune response to HIV may help the treatment of those who already have AIDS.

Once the vaccine is prepared, it must go through "phases" before it can be used on the public. Phase I trials determine whether the "candidate" vaccine is safe and does not have unacceptable side effects. These studies will employ small numbers of healthy adult volunteers. An evaluation of the immune response in these volunteers will also be made.

Phase II trials involve larger numbers of volunteers, including persons at high risk of infection with HIV. These trials are designed to determine an optimal dosage regimen with respect to safety and immune response.

Phase III trials evaluate the capacity of the candidate vaccine to protect against disease and provide further knowledge about its safety. These trials are generally randomized, placebo controlled, and double-blind. The sample size is based upon the incidence of infection in the study population and the level of statistical certainty that researchers determine is sufficient to protect from infection and disease.

More Problems With the AIDS Vaccine

There are problems with the development of a vaccine for HIV that are particular, if not unique. 1) The virus has a latent period of several years, even decades, between infection and manifestation of disease. The average period from time of infection with HIV until the presence of AIDS is almost 10 years. The efficacy of a vaccine, then, may have to be evaluated against *prevention of infection* rather than protection against disease *after infection* because the latter would take almost a decade to determine its efficacy.

2) Those vaccinated will test positive to the ELISA, the common screening test for the presence of HIV, because they will have antibodies that cause that test to react positively. While other tests could be employed to prove that they were not infected with HIV, it easy to see how their lives would be complicated by these positive tests.

3) HIV is one of the most rapidly mutating viruses known. Any one person infected with it commonly has several genetically different strains at any one time and in different parts of his body.[3] One vaccine is not likely to be effective against all these strains.

4) HIV does not infect animals, so there are no suitable

animal models in which to test this vaccine. Artificially infected mouse models have been developed, but the applicability of research with them to humans has not been determined. The chimpanzee becomes infected with HIV, but it does not produce an AIDS-like illness.

"Speaking of Other Things" Relative to All Vaccines

The liability status of all vaccines is currently in question. Lawsuits over the complications of some vaccines have caused many manufacturers to stop making them altogether. Liability insurance accounts for some 90 percent of the current cost of vaccines. If an AIDS vaccine is developed, the federal government will have to prohibit or severely limit liability awards. Otherwise, no private company will market it because the potential cost for a complication would be astronomical.

It almost seems sacrilegious (relative to "orthodox" medicine) to mention, but the issue of efficacy for all vaccines is still questionable. Disability and death from many prevalent diseases of the past (for example, polio and smallpox) had decreased markedly *before* the widespread use of vaccines against them.[4] Yet, because the timing was coincidental, the vaccine and "modern medicine" gets the credit!

Further, vaccines are not without their unintended effects, some of which can be fatal. All vaccines need to be closely and extensively researched as to their overall impact on disease. To my knowledge, this comprehensive study has not yet been done.

The Moral (Biblical) Considerations

For the discussion here, all people are divided into three groups according to the context of their risk. The first group is the population at large who is extremely unlikely to be exposed to HIV. The second group consists of those who are married with an intention to live their lifetime with one spouse, but who also have a probability of exposure: persons with spouses who have HIV, medical personnel who work with AIDS patients, and children born to mothers with HIV. The third group are those who practice the confirmed high-risk practices for HIV infection: fornication, adultery, homosexuality, and IV-drug abuse.

Whether to develop a vaccine for the first group is debatable. This group has virtually no risk of infection with HIV. The primary factor in this decision depends upon one's belief that the virus may mutate in a way that causes it to become infectious by casual routes. I do not think that it will, but I would support the development of a vaccine for this purpose, since the process will likely take a decade or more. If the virus does mutate, it will be too late to begin the vaccine process after mutation has occurred.

The second group has the clearest reason for the development of the vaccine. They are the innocent (of moral cause-and-effect) victims of this epidemic. Their plight alone is sufficient reason to develop the vaccine. However, the unborn can benefit only by their mothers' becoming vaccinated before they become pregnant.

The third group wants a vaccine in order to continue to practice their immorality without the specter of AIDS. They want to be protected from this consequence of their sin. It is my contention that this motive is morally wrong.

The Biblical principle is that God does not call us to assist others to avoid the consequences of their sin. Further, it is sin for us to assist them in this way. "And do not participate in the unfruitful deeds of darkness, but instead even expose them" (Ephesians 5:11, NASB).

The situation can be posed this way. Will the removal of the consequences of HIV infection promote either physical or spiritual health over the long term? While a vaccine may prevent this one disease, the sexually immoral will be exposed to many other sexually transmitted diseases over their lifetimes. Further, they will be worsening their spiritual condition. That is, their entrenchment in their sin will become worse. (Biblically, their hearts will become more hardened.)

A vaccine for HIV has the same moral perspective as the prescription of birth control pills by physicians to unmarried women.[5] Studies have shown that the prescription of birth control pills actually causes an increase in the problems that they are supposed to prevent: frequency of sexual intercourse and the rate of illegitimate pregnancy. More frequent sexual intercourse increases the likelihood of infection with a sexually transmitted disease. An increase in pregnancies is more likely to result in abortion (the primary "good" that physicians often give as an excuse to prescribe birth control to these women).

After all, you see, *God did build this universe and the human race*. He designed physical laws to govern the physical universe and spiritual laws to govern man's behavior. The unity of His Person requires that both the physical and spiritual dimensions be consistent. Thus, violations of the law of gravity will cause injury and death. Violations of laws of spirituality (e.g., "Thou shalt not commit adultery") will cause injury and death.

God would also be inconsistent to allow man's design of physical tools (the practice of medicine) to be able to overcome His spiritual laws. Thus, *to expect medicine to be able to limit the consequences of sin is incompatible with God's very nature.* In spite of the best medical care ever available to mankind, we still have the modern epidemics of sexually transmitted diseases and AIDS.

Thus, my only expectation of an AIDS vaccine that is made available to those who want to be protected from the consequences of their sin is *that the epidemic of AIDS will actually increase, or a worse sexually transmitted disease may appear*! It is not so hard to understand. If the threat of AIDS is minimized, then promiscuity and sexual perversion will only get worse, resulting in an escalation of an already-severe problem.

Another moral question is "How much money should be spent by the federal government on research for an AIDS vaccine?" It does seems reasonable that the amount of money spent on a vaccine should be proportional to the prevalence and incidence of HIV and AIDS in the population and on projected estimates of future numbers. I see no reason that research for this disease should take priority over that of other diseases. In fact, I can see good reasons why it should not, namely, those practices that are high risk are immoral, illegal, or both.

A vaccine for AIDS, then, should be developed to protect the "innocents" who will be exposed to HIV and for the possibility that HIV may mutate and become infectious by casual exposure. It is Biblically wrong to develop a vaccine to prevent the consequences of sinful behavior for those who are guilty.

Conclusions

While you and I may have little or no effect on plans for an AIDS vaccine, we should understand the technical and moral issues. Likely, more research and money will be spent on this endeavor than has been spent on any single medical problem in our nation's history. The goal of that research is primarily to preserve the same practices that caused this epidemic in the first place! Does not that sort of reasoning strike you as pouring fuel on a fire?

A vaccine may be developed, and probably should be, but the root problem of sexual immorality (within a secular worldview) has not been acknowledged. Until it is, sexually transmitted diseases will continue in epidemic proportions with the possibility of worse diseases than AIDS. In God's universe, the physical and the spiritual are intimately linked in a way that is consistent with His own Person and Unity.

> "Do not be deceived, God is not mocked; for whatever a man sows, this he will also reap. For the one who sows to his own flesh shall from the flesh reap corruption, but the one who sows to the Spirit shall from the Spirit reap eternal life" (Galatians 6:7-8, NASB).

A New Development

Vaccines are usually given to prevent infections. One exception is vaccination against rabies that is begun *after* a bite-exposure of a human to a rabid animal. Recently published research, however, suggests that vaccination against HIV may be effective *after infection.*[6]

Dr. Robert Redfield and his colleagues found that their vaccine prevented a decline in those cells most affected by

HIV, the CD4 cells (a type of T-cell), in patients already infected with HIV. While their research was a Phase I trial and clinical effects are supposed to be measured in Phase II and/or Phase III, these results suggest that vaccines may be effective after infection with HIV has occurred.

Notes and References

1. A "germ" may be a virus, a bacterium, a parasite, or other invading organism. Antibodies are developed primarily against viruses and bacteria.

2. Wayne C. Koff and Daniel F. Hoth, "Development and Testing of AIDS Vaccines," *Science* 241 (July 22, 1988):426-432.

3. Jon Van, "AIDS Virus Shown to Evolve Greatly in Body," *Chicago Tribune* (June 13, 1991), Section 1, 10.

4. Leonard A. Sagan, *The Health of Nations: True Causes of Sickness and Well-Being* (New York: Basic Books, Inc., 1987), 28-41.

5. Barrett L. Mosbacker, "Promiscuity, Prophylactics, and the Christian Physician," *Journal of Biblical Ethics in Medicine* 2 (October 1988):68-74.

6. Robert R. Redfield, "A Phase I Evaluation of the Safety and Immunogenicity of Vaccination With Recombinant gp160 in Patients With Early Human Immunodeficiency Virus Infection," *The New England Journal of Medicine* 324 (June 13, 1991):1677-1684.

CHAPTER 14

Winning the War Against AIDS: Our Nation's Response vs. A Biblical Response

by Herbert W. Titus, J.D.[1]

Writing in the August 1985 *Journal of the Royal Society of Medicine*, Dr. John Seale, an infectious disease expert, has warned that AIDS (Acquired Immune Deficiency Syndrome) is a plague capable of producing "a lethal pandemic throughout crowded cities and villages of the Third World of a magnitude unparalleled in human history."[2]

Despite the threat of such a devastating plague, Christians have hope in their Lord, Jesus Christ. They have hope in the mercy of God, revealed through the Word of God. While we rest in this hope and continue to proclaim it to the world, we should also understand the present conditions concerning AIDS and our nation's response to it.

A Legal Revolution Has Occurred

These conditions would not have been possible had it not been for a virtual legal revolution in the 1960s and 70s. The changes which occurred went largely unnoticed by the Church. The revolution came through the wholesale change of the criminal laws of various states. These states accepted the recommendations made by the American Law Institute in its acclaimed Model Penal Code. The Code was sponsored by lawyers and judges in an effort to reform and standardize criminal law throughout the nation. Included were provisions that would repeal laws against adultery, homosexual behavior, bestiality, and other laws that prohibited private sexual activity outside the bonds of marriage.

These proposals were based upon the assumption that private sexual practices between consenting adults threaten no harm to the community. This viewpoint was first supported by an official government report from Great Britain in 1957.[3] Criminal law experts in the United States popularized recommendations from the report through a plethora of articles and books. It was claimed that private consensual adult sexual offenses were "victimless crimes." This idea was widely accepted as the Model Penal Code reforms were presented to various state legislatures in the 1960s and 70s. *To the disgrace of the Christian community*, few voices were raised against the repeal of the traditional laws prohibiting fornication, adultery, sodomy, and bestiality.

With the outbreak of AIDS and other incurable sexually transmitted diseases, the American people are awakening to realize that unchecked sexual promiscuity threatens not only its participants, but all of society. Yet they have been opposed by the same experts who pushed for the liberalization of the laws. Despite overwhelming evidence to the contrary, many of America's political leaders, legal and medical experts, and religious leaders have been unwilling to admit that they were mistaken about the dangers of the sexual revolution they helped to foster.

These leaders have put faith in the ability of medical experts to discover "cures" for AIDS and other venereal diseases. They look to science as the standard-setter for public policy. In the meantime, they have resisted most efforts to protect the American populace from the threat of contamination. They fear that by doing so, they would concede that private sexual acts of traditional immorality, committed by consenting adults were, after all, *not* "victimless crimes."

Biblical Roots for American Law

Why have America's leaders strayed so far? The answer is simple. They have rejected Biblical foundations for law and, therefore, the order and security upon which the American nation has prospered for over 375 years. Had America's leaders kept the faith of her founders, they would never have supported the repeal of the criminal laws prohibiting adultery, fornication, sodomy, and bestiality.

In 1798, Jesse Root, a leading member of the Connecticut Bar and a respected lawyer throughout the United States, wrote that the Bible was America's "Magna Charta."[4] Drawing from their knowledge of Biblical principles, America's political and legal state founded a system of criminal laws that both ensured order and guaranteed liberty.

Unchecked sexual activity was not afforded the protection of law, because God had revealed it to be contrary to the "laws of nature," that is, contrary to the law of the nature of man whom God had created. The homosexual act, for example, was called a "crime against nature" in America until the last twenty or twenty-five years. Had this view prevailed in law and in practice in America, this nation would not be faced with the AIDS explosion today.

A Three-Fold Biblical Response

Even so, all is not lost. America has not been left without an effective remedy. But her leaders must return to the Bible that has served the nation for so long. The Bible directs a three-fold response to the AIDS plague. First, AIDS must be recognized as a medical problem. Many innocent people have already been infected, and many more are threatened. In Leviticus 13, God has given guidelines designed to protect the innocent from the threat of contagious diseases such as AIDS. This traditional response has been used in America and in nations around the world. It involves the isolation and quarantine of those who are *suspected* of having a contagious or infectious disease.[5]

God has authorized the appropriate civil officials, even before there is a determination that a disease is infectious or contagious, to find and quarantine those already infected. (See Chapter 11.) They must not wait until it has been determined that the disease is infectious before a quarantine is put into effect. To the contrary, they should find and quarantine first.

Only after proper studies have clearly determined that the disease is *not* contagious or infectious should the diseased populace be allowed to mingle freely in society. Otherwise, the civil authorities have not done their duty to protect innocent people from a potentially serious threat of physical harm. (See Romans 13:4.)

The primary purpose of this Biblical health policy is to protect the public from contamination. Persons who are suspected of carrying infectious or contagious diseases are required to surrender some of their personal freedoms, at least temporarily, for the good of the community at large. The personal rights and liberties of infected individuals (or even those suspected of being infected) always come second to the physical health and welfare of the whole community.

This requirement does not mean that those who are infected have engaged in sinful practices. Rather it is for the medical purposes of cleanliness and isolation, designed to protect the general population from physical contamination. Proper health policy for a fatal, communicable disease such as AIDS is not a matter of prejudice against homosexuals or any other group. It is simply a matter of the civil authorities fulfilling their duty to protect the healthy populace from a contagious, killer disease.

Second, no medical problem can be resolved without an examination to determine if it is the consequence of sin. Jesus Christ taught that some diseases or physical defects are *not* the direct consequence of personal sin. (See John 9:1-3.) But God has also revealed that sometimes people are afflicted with disease because of specific misdeeds. In regard to the practice of homosexuality, this connection is suggested in Romans 1:27. The high incidence of AIDS among today's homosexuals confirms that, indeed, AIDS is not only a medical problem, but also a sin problem.

Whenever there is a close connection between sin and disease, a society's religious leaders are called to intercede on behalf of those who have suffered from their own folly. For example, Moses cried out to God to heal his sister Miriam after she had been afflicted with leprosy for her rebellious behavior. (See Numbers 12:13.) Because of Moses' intercession, Miriam was healed.

Intercession may be required for an entire nation. The people of Israel murmured and grumbled against Aaron and Moses after God quieted the rebellion of Korah. (See Numbers 16:41.) As a consequence, the entire nation was threatened by a "consuming plague." Moses and Aaron hastily made atonement to God on the nation's behalf. As Aaron "took his stand between the dead and the living...the plague was checked." (See Numbers 16:48.)

In II Samuel 24, the Bible teaches that a plague had come upon the people of Israel as a direct consequence of King David's personal sin. David wept because he realized that his sin had caused a disease to come upon innocent people. With a heart of repentance, he built an altar, offered a sacrifice, and prayed for the people. God answered David's prayers on behalf of the land, and He stopped the plague. (See II Samuel 24:25.)

Such intercession by a nation's religious leaders is necessary to invoke God's mercy upon the land. Also, appropriate action by the leaders should influence those who are sinning to repent and to receive God's forgiveness. Without intercession by the leaders and without a response from the people, the "law of the land," as revealed in the Bible, will respond to the sin that is polluting the nation. The nation's inhabitants will suffer destructions of various kinds. Eventually, it is written, the land will "vomit out" its corrupted inhabitants. (See Leviticus 18:26-28.) Continual violation of the laws of nature, without intercession and repentance, will lead any nation to destruction.

If a disease, or the spread of a disease, is the direct consequence of sin, medical treatment alone will not solve the problem. Permanent relief will truly be forthcoming only as the mercy of God is sought and the transgression is forsaken. But if the people have hardened their hearts to a sin problem and have allowed the sin to flourish in the land, the nation not only faces a sin problem, but also a crime problem.

Third, AIDS is unmistakably a crime problem in America. Homosexuals have been allowed to practice their sin freely without accountability to Biblical standards enforceable by civil society. Indeed, they have been encouraged to engage in sinful sexual practices as if they had a "right" to do so without discrimination or other penalty.

However, the fact that homosexual practices have largely been "decriminalized" throughout the nation does not make such behavior any less a crime. Upon examination of the Bible, the following truth becomes clear: It is false to assume that private, promiscuous sexual activity among consenting adults has no victims.

God created woman for man and ordained marriage, a lifelong commitment, as the only acceptable avenue for sexual relationships. (See Genesis 2:24.) He did not create the male sex to have sexual relations with men nor the female sex to have sexual relations with women. All homosexual activity, therefore, is contrary to the very nature of man.

God has warned that unchecked perversion in sexual relations will inevitably bring harm to the participants *and to the society that tolerates it*. All nations are warned that if homosexual behavior and bestiality are tolerated, their land will be "defiled." (See Leviticus 18:22-29.)

In other words, homosexual activity is *not*, according to the Bible, a "victimless crime." To the contrary, such perverse sexual activity, even if accomplished in private by consenting adults, is a crime that defiles the land and endangers the security of the nation.

This state of affairs may be illustrated by another incident that occurred early in the history of Israel. In Numbers 25, the Bible has recorded a time when the people openly engaged in sexual immorality in defiance of their families, their society, and their God. As a consequence, a "plague" came upon the people. The plague continued unchecked until one of Israel's leaders punished two of the most serious offenders. (See Numbers 25:8.) Because civil justice for the commission of a crime was administered, God spared Israel from destruction. (See Psalm 106:30-31.)

In summary, the Bible teaches a three-fold response to a contagious plague such as AIDS. First, steps must be taken immediately to isolate and to quarantine those infected in order to afford medical protection to the public. Second, intercessions must be made on behalf of the nation and of those involved in any sin connected with the plague. Those involved in homosexual sin must be encouraged to repent and seek forgiveness from God. Finally, the civil rulers must identify those who choose to defy laws which prohibit homosexuality. Such laws must be retained in each state and enforced. Special attention should be given to those who lead others into open and habitual practice of homosexuality and other illicit sexual acts.

Recent Secular Responses

Recent responses to AIDS in our nation have failed to secure the protection of society afforded by a Biblical response. First, consider the policy of United States Public Health officials. On January 26, 1984, Margaret Heckler, then Secretary of Health and Human Services, made a speech before the U.S. Conference of Mayors AIDS Task Force. She claimed that the "first task" was to inform and educate the public so as to disabuse it of a plague mentality.[6] Because of that policy, federal health officials have been encouraged to concentrate *not* on how best to protect the public from what is apparently a deadly contagious and infectious disease. Rather, the emphasis has been placed upon what can be done to relieve those who suffer from AIDS.

Spokesmen for the Centers for Disease Control (CDC) have consistently reassured the American public that blood contamination and sexual contact appear to be the only means of transmission, while other researchers are more cautious, because "body fluids and excretions from AIDS patients, such as saliva, tears, urine, and feces, are also considered to be possibly infectious."[7]

Such discoveries have led ophthalmologists to change their procedures in order to avoid contact with the AIDS virus that may be in the tears of AIDS patients. Other professionals have taken similar precautions. Doctors John Sensakovic and Benjamin Greer, authors of an article written for health-care personnel, have made the following recommendations for handling AIDS patients:

> "A private room is probably desirable, if for no other reason than to act as a reminder of the importance of isolation techniques. If the patient is unable to maintain good hygiene, a private room is mandatory. Gowns, gloves, and scrupulous hand washing are essential. Masks are not necessary, unless there is a possibility that the patient's saliva will be sprayed into the air... Where there is any risk of spraying or splashing of infectious materials, protective eye coverings should also be used." [8]

The same authors advise fire and first-aid personnel that "direct mouth-to-mouth resuscitation should be avoided with known AIDS patients."[9]

Three other medical instructors from the University of Medicine and Dentistry of New Jersey-Rutgers Medical School, have written, "Although there is no evidence that AIDS may be transmitted in saliva, the concern about mouth-to-mouth resuscitation is probably valid because there may be blood in the patient's mouth."[10]

Yet when parents ask for protection for their children in the public schools, many school officials, politicians, lawyers, and government health officials insist that there is *no* danger. They say that children with AIDS should be allowed to attend regular classes. It is ironic that parents are required to send their children to school with students who have AIDS but are prohibited from sending them to school if they do not have their tuberculin skin test.

Newt Gingrich, a U.S. Representative from Georgia, warns that few public health officials are aware of the rising public anxiety over the AIDS epidemic. "Prudent behavior historically would be to seal off the disease, find a cure, and then relax. The public health bureaucracy wants to relax first, then seal off the disease, then find a cure."[11] A close look at government activity in the AIDS matter suggests, however, that Gingrich is not quite accurate. The public health bureaucracy has sought to find a cure first, before sealing off the disease.

Paul Weyrich suggests a reason for this backward health policy: "The public senses a very deep problem, one where their safety and welfare are threatened, but the politicians have been scared because the homosexual lobby, like the civil rights lobby, has exaggerated importance in Washington."[12]

There is another reason why America's public health officials have failed to respond in a sensible, Biblical way with respect to AIDS as a medical problem. They fear even the suggestion that AIDS is related to a sin problem: "Appearing to be unenlightened,...the public health intelligentsia, in common with the organized homosexuals, still clings to the dogma that 'you can't legislate morality' and claims that legal discrimination against homosexuality is irrational--'homophobia'--and a 'return to the Dark Ages.'"[13]

In an effort to encourage the recognition of homosexuality and heterosexuality as morally equal, America's leaders have confused their priorities in addressing AIDS as a medical problem. As a result, thousands of innocent people may suffer.

What is the recent response to AIDS as a sin problem? A pamphlet circulated among colleges and universities describes the dominant approach to AIDS on the nation's campuses. In it, the American College Health Association has endorsed the view that homosexual behavior is not wrong: "Don't mistake a recommendation of caution for a condemnation of homosexuality or of sexual expression."[14] In other words, America's college and university health officials have denied even the possibility that there may be a sin problem underlying the outbreak of AIDS.

Therefore, they have advised students to lessen their risk of contracting AIDS by taking halfway precautions such as: "Reducing your number of sexual partners"; "showering before and after sex"; and "curtailing the use of illicit drugs."[15]

Because the nation's educational authorities are unwilling to deal with AIDS as a sin problem, those calling for repentance from the nation's pulpits face a serious uphill battle.

Concerning AIDS as a crime problem, some civil authorities have chosen to legalize and protect homosexual activity even at the expense of the public's health and life. Already many cities and local communities have enacted ordinances to guarantee homosexuals the right to practice their lifestyle openly without fear of discrimination in housing or employment. Bolstered by such victories, homosexual "civil rights" groups have insisted on similar legal protection for those with AIDS.

For example, on August 14, 1985, the Los Angeles City Council passed an ordinance that makes it a crime to discriminate against persons with AIDS in the areas of employment, housing and health care.[16] Only blood and sperm banks are exempted. Employment decisions in businesses such as hotels, restaurants, dentistry and medicine are especially affected. The potential threat that an employee could transmit the AIDS virus to a patient or customer cannot be taken into account.

For example, a dentist, concerned for the health of his patients and knowing the uncertainties that surround the transmission of the AIDS virus, is well aware of the fact that blood and saliva are unavoidable elements in a dental hygienist's daily work. However, he would violate the city ordinance if he dismisses an AIDS-infected dental hygienist. Ironically, the Los Angeles city officials have decided to protect those who may have contracted AIDS because of their wrongful sexual activities, even though they pose a direct threat to others who are innocent of such wrongdoing.

Conclusion

Why has America come to this? What has occurred in this great nation, now that its leaders call evil "good" and good "evil"? America is a nation that began with the Bible as its legal and political Magna Charta. How has it departed so far from that charter in its failure to respond appropriately to the AIDS epidemic which threatens its security and prosperity?

The answer may be found in a letter written by the apostle Paul to the Church in first-century Rome. At the time Paul wrote, the Roman Empire tolerated sexual promiscuity in the same way twentieth-century America does. Paul explained that Roman society had become that way because it was dominated by the thinking of men who denied that man had been created in the image of God. (See Romans 1:22-25.)

Indeed, this was the case. One century before Christ, a

man named Lucretius wrote a book to support those who chose to live a life of pleasure without concern for divine judgment. In his book *On the Nature of Things*,[17] Lucretius subscribed to an evolutionary faith. He wrote that the world and man had originated via a "big bang," and consequently, are governed by the law of "survival of the fittest." Such thinking led men to justify all kinds of perverse sexual activity, although contrary to man's very nature. (See Romans 1:26-27.)

In America's schools today, the Roman theory of evolution dominates the classrooms. For two or three generations, her children have been taught that man evolved by time and chance from lower forms of animals. Considering the words of Paul, it has been no accident that homosexual activity has increased in America. For under such instruction, man has become a fool, having "exchanged the glory of the incorruptible God for an image in the form of four-footed animals and crawling creatures. Therefore, God gave them over in the lusts of their hearts to impurity, that their bodies might be dishonored among them" (Romans 1:23-24).

America is reaping what she has sown. (See Galatians 6:7.) Our nation must respond in a Biblical way to the AIDS plague. A Biblical response in no way warrants a hate campaign against homosexuals or any other group, but it does necessitate three steps of action. First, the AIDS problem must be treated in a medically sane way. The health and welfare of the general population must be given higher priority than the so-called civil liberties of those infected with the fatal and communicable disease. Second, America must acknowledge that homosexuality is more than a "victimless crime." It is a wrong that affects all of society. Third, our civil authorities must reenact and enforce laws that define illicit sexual behavior as a crime. Those who persist in practicing such behavior must be prosecuted.

If our nation fails to respond according to the laws of the Creator, we will be inviting more depravity, and even ultimate destruction, upon our land.

Notes and References

1. Dr. Titus is Provost and Dean, College of Law and Government, Regent University, Virginia Beach, Virginia.

2. Quoted in Richard Restak, "Society's Survival First, Then Victims' Rights," *Human Events* (October 5, 1985):19. Dr. Seale's prediction has come true, as HIV/AIDS is devastating Africa and other Third World countries.

3. Congressional Research Service, Issue Brief, IB83162, Updated March 4, 1985, reported in "AIDS--The Gay Plague and 'Civil Rights,'" *Eye on Bureaucracy*, published by the Conservative Caucus Research, Analysis and Education Foundation (June 1985):1.

4. "Home Office Scottish Home Department Report on the Committee on Homosexual Offenses and Prostitution" (Wolfenden Report), quoted in part in Monrad G. Paulsen and Sanford H. Kadish, *Criminal Law and Its Processes: Cases and Materials* (Boston and Toronto: Little, Brown and Company, 1962), 5-8.

5. Perry Miller, ed., *The Legal Mind in America, From Independence to the Civil War* (Ithaca, New York: Cornell University Press, 1962), 34-36.

6. Reported in "AIDS--The Gay Plague and 'Civil Rights,'" *Eye on Bureaucracy* (June 1985): 4.

7. John W. Sensakovic and Benjamin Greer, "Preventing AIDS," in *Understanding AIDS: A Comprehensive Guide*, ed. Victor Gong (New Brunswick, New Jersey: Rutgers University Press, 1985), 168.

8. *Ibid.*

9. *Ibid.*, 171.

10. Victor Gong, Michael Marsh and Daniel Shindler, "Questions and Answers about AIDS," in *Understanding AIDS: A Comprehensive Guide*, ed. Victor Gong, (New Brunswick, New Jersey: Rutgers University Press, 1985), 198.

11. Quoted in Fred Barnes, "The Politics of AIDS," *The New Republic* (November 4, 1985):12.

12. *Ibid.*

13. John Adams Wettergreen, "AIDS, Public Morality, and Public Health," *Claremont Review of Books* (Fall 1985):5.

14. Quoted in Lawrence Biemiller, "AIDS on Campus: Concern Goes Beyond Health as Officials Prepare to Handle a Flood of Questions," *The Chronicle of Higher Education* 31 (October 2, 1985):40.

15. *Ibid.*

16. Restak, "Society's Survival First, Then Victims' Rights," 18.

17. Lucretius, *On the Nature of Things*, trans. Charles E. Bennet (Roslyn, New York: Walter J. Black, Inc., 1946), 231-298.

APPENDIX

A Comparative Analysis of the Risk of HIV in Health-Care Workers: Implications for Hospital Policy[1]

Jane M. Orient, M.D.[2]

Hospital infection control committees grappling with the problem of protecting health-care workers against human immunodeficiency virus (HIV) face a number of unresolved legal and ethical issues.

One viewpoint is that the most important problem is the potential stigma faced by HIV-positive patients. To protect such patients against emotional distress and the possibility of discrimination should their status become known, the hospitals require specific written informed consent for HIV testing. Various medical organizations have made policy statements that may establish this requirement as the standard of care,[3] despite the fact that specific consent forms were used by only 27.5 percent of 187 U.S. hospitals having training programs in infectious diseases, and were usually not mandatory.[4]

The Occupational Safety and Health Administration (OSHA) requires that workers be informed of risks: e.g., "Biological hazard tags shall be used to identify the actual or potential presence of a biological hazard and to identify equipment, containers, rooms, experimental animals, or combinations thereof, that contain or are contaminated with hazardous biological agents."[5] To comply with this directive, hospitals have adopted "universal precautions," informing workers that *any* patient *might* be HIV positive.

It is frequently stated that medical work has always been hazardous, and that those who undertake it freely accept all the attendant risks. (In this sense, AIDS is considered to be the *same* as tuberculosis, plague, and other infectious diseases; however, it is *different* in the sense that ordering diagnostic tests, labeling specimens, and placing isolation signs may be contraindicated for AIDS, while required for tuberculosis, varicella zoster, hepatitis, etc.) In any event, the risk of acquiring AIDS from caring for afflicted patients is said to be "slight" (even after the most careless of exposures),[6] "extremely small,"[7] or "low."[8] Seminars are scheduled to help workers overcome their fears.[9]

Missing from the exhortations to become comfortable with AIDS is an effort to compare the risks with those of other occupational hazards.

How "Low" is the Likelihood of AIDS Transmission From a Needlestick?

Needlesticks are a common occupational injury and may constitute the most important risk event for health-care workers. The risk that a health-care worker will be infected with HIV as a result of a single needlestick is given by: $P_{i,hcw} = (P_{i,\ pt})(P_{t})$, where $P_{i,\ hcw}$ is the probability of infection being transmitted to the health-care worker, $P_{i,pt}$ is the probability that the source patient is infected, and P_t is the conditional probability that transmission (as manifested by seroconversion) will occur, given that the patient is infected.

Obviously, if the patient is not infected, the probability of HIV transmission is zero. If the patient is known to be infected, then $P_{i,pt} = 1$. In that instance, if P_t is taken to be 0.35 percent (upper confidence limit 0.90 percent),[10] then the risk of seroconversion due to a single needlestick is 0.35 percent or 0.0035. If the prevalence of seropositivity in the population is 1 in 1000, then a needlestick from a known positive source exposes the health-care worker to 1000-times as great a risk as a needlestick from a source patient randomly selected from that population.

To calculate the risk that a health-care worker will seroconvert as a result of a single procedure using a needle in a seropositive patient, one must know the frequency of needlestick injuries. One center reported a rate of 1.9 needlesticks per 1000 HIV-positive patient days in 1986, a decrease from 4.6 in 1984.[11] Assuming that 2 procedures involving a needle are done per average patient day, one can estimate that the risk of a stick on a given procedure is about 1 in 1000, or 0.1 percent. This would give a risk per procedure (in 1986) of 3.5×10^{-6}.

Another method of calculating the rate of needlestick injuries is to consider the number of reported sticks per 100,000 items purchased. The rate was 18.4 per 100,000 for intravenous catheters with stylets; 25.4 per 100,000 for vacuum-tube phlebotomy assemblies; and 36.7 per 100,000 for intravenous tubing/needle assemblies.[12] These figures would give a seroconversion risk per procedure of 6.4×10^{-7}, 8.89×10^{-7}, and 12.8×10^{-7}, respectively.

The risk of performing a single procedure involving a needle puncture is, thus, quite small. However, AIDS patients are likely to require a large number of needle punctures. The probability that *no* health-care worker will seroconvert in performing 1000 needle punctures is calculated from the binomial probability distribution: $P_{0,1000} = (P_{i,hcw})^0 (P_{ni,\ hcw})^{1000}$, where P_{ni}, the probability that the worker will *not* convert on one given procedure, is $(1 - P_{i,hcw})$.

The probability that at least one worker *will* seroconvert in the performance of 1000 procedures is $(1 - P_{0,1000})$. The probabilities as calculated from the above assumptions are given in Table 1, along with the annual risk of death due to certain other occupations. The probability of infection will be correspondingly higher if the rate of needlesticks is under reported, as has been the case previously,[13] or if the rate of HIV transmission is higher. (Using the upper confidence limit of 0.9 percent for the rate of disease transmission due to a single contaminated needlestick, the risk increases to 165-896 in 100,000.)

Table 1

Occupational Risks

Occupational hazard	Per 100,000*
HIV seroconversion+	64-349@
Policemen killed in line of duty[14]	22
All industrial deaths[15]	15
Construction deaths[16]	60
Mining and quarrying deaths[17]	66
Death on Louisiana oil rig[18]	188-283
"Acceptable" occupational risk[19]	10
Natural-hazards mortality rate#	0.1

* Annual
\+ Due to performing needle punctures on HIV-positive patients
@ Per 1000 procedures
\# Defined as "low" or "trivial" rate[20]

The rate of seroconversion from a single needlestick (P_t) may be underestimated if the time to seroconversion is longer than one year (especially in cases with a small inoculum). Attributing seropositivity in a health-care worker to another risk factor whenever one can be identified may also cause underestimation of the occupational risk.

If the assumptions concerning the risk of needlestick injuries are correct, then performing 1000 needle punctures on HIV-positive patients (say an average of 3 daily for 333 days) may be more dangerous than a year of work on a Louisiana oil rig, one of the most hazardous occupations currently available. Doing a smaller number of procedures is approximately as dangerous as working on the oil rig for a corresponding fraction of a year. As with all occupational injuries, workers of greater experience and skill may be at less risk.

For surgeons, the risk is much higher than for other health-care workers. It has been estimated that a surgeon experiences parenteral exposure to blood once in 43 operations, on the average.[21] Using the same risk of transmission as above (0.0035), the probability that a surgeon will seroconvert *as a result of one operation* on a seropositive patient is 0.0000814 (8.14 in 100,000, nearly the "acceptable" occupational risk for a full year). The risk of becoming seropositive is 7.8 percent (7800 in 100,000) after 1000 such operations, and 33 percent after 5000 operations.

In actuality, the death rate from occupationally transmitted HIV may be much higher than from oil-rig accidents because workers infected with HIV can infect their spouses, their unborn children, and others. In one study, 23 percent of 97 female sexual partners of HIV-positive men were also seropositive.[22] In another, 58 percent of 45 spouses were seropositive.[23] Updated results from the latter study (after a median follow-up of 18 months) showed HIV antibodies present in 17 percent of spouses who used condoms and in 82 percent of those who did not, while continuing sexual activity.[24] (There were only 18 couples in the group using condoms. The upper confidence limit for the percentage converting in this length of time is approximately 40 percent.) In the 12 couples who practiced abstinence after the diagnosis was made, there were no seroconversions. Thus, for monogamous health-care workers who continue sexual relations after an exposure to HIV, the risk given in Table 1 should be increased, probably by 20 percent at least. For health-care workers who have more than one sexual partner, the public health effects of exposure to HIV are vastly greater. If one person infects one other person per year, and each of the infected contacts also transmits the disease to one person per year, there would be 1024 cases (2^{10}) at the end of 10 years.

Managing the Risk of HIV Transmission

It is imperative to reduce the rate of needlestick injuries. One study estimated that 40 percent of needlesticks are theoretically preventable (outside the operating room) by following recommended precautions, e.g., for proper handling and disposal of needles.[25] One method is to forbid the recapping of needles, because one-third of all the injuries were related to this practice.[26] However, it has yet to be shown that the injury rate can be reduced by as much as one-third in this way. Often, health-care workers report that the reason for recapping the needle is the perception of a competing hazard.

Other suggested precautions include the development of novel methods that do not require the use of needles: devices that allow the needle to remain covered during and after use, and puncture-resistant gloves. Double gloving has also been recommended, based upon evidence that latex gloves contain holes larger than the virus,[27] although the significance of this finding has been disputed.[28] Surgeons might slow down, avoid the use of electrocautery and wire sutures,[29] pick up instruments themselves, and approach certain intracranial lesions via stereotactic biopsy instead of open craniotomy.[30] Implementation of these methods will certainly carry a monetary price, as well as a loss in efficiency and manual dexterity. Already, one Tucson hospital spends $300,000 annually for "universal precautions" of gloves and gowns.[31]

The prevention of all needlesticks would not completely eliminate the risk of infection. Of 15 well-documented, published cases of infection due to occupational events (in which no non-occupational risk could be identified), 5 did not involve needlesticks or cuts with sharp objects.[32] Personnel working with high-risk patients or specimens might wish to use additional barrier precautions such as masks and goggles to prevent contact of blood with skin or mucous membranes. Laboratory workers might choose to use screw-cap centrifuge cups, save high-risk specimens for the end of the run, just prior to work-surface disinfection, or take other extraordinary precautions.[33]

Once a health-care worker does suffer a needlestick injury or other exposure, how should the hospital respond? The worker can be offered serial tests. But what counseling should be given while the worker is awaiting the results of tests scheduled as far as six months and one year into the future, with the knowledge that an infected person may transmit disease to others before seroconversion occurs?

Potential courses of action include sexual abstinence for a period of time (up to six months or more), the use of condoms (which do, however, have a failure rate estimated to be as high as 17 percent,[34]) and prescription of zidovudine,[35] despite the lack of proven benefit, with the attendant toxicity and expense.

In order to make an informed decision, most health-care workers will want very much to know whether or not the source patient was infected. If the patient is not infected, the health-care worker need not choose between placing his loved ones at risk (albeit somewhat less than his or her own), an action that could be severely disruptive of his or her home life. The worker and loved ones would all be spared mental anguish.

Of course, there is the possibility of a false negative test in the source patient. The likelihood of a false negative varies with the prevalence and incidence of disease in the patient population, and is estimated to be about 2-3 in 10,000 if the prevalence of disease is 1 percent, assuming that the test has a sensitivity of 99 percent and that it takes 6 weeks to develop antibodies after infection has occurred.[36] Thus, in such populations, a negative result lowers the risk that the source patient is infected by a factor of about 40, compared with the risk from an unknown source. (The prior probability is 0.01 and the posterior probability, between 0.0002 and 0.0003.) Many health-care workers might perceive that to be a difference large enough to affect their decisions. If the prevalence of disease is 5 percent and the annual incidence is 1 percent, a negative test lowers the probability of infection in the source patient from 0.05 to 0.0017, i.e., by a factor of 29.

There is also the possibility of a false positive test, causing needless anxiety in both the patient and the exposed worker. However, a very low rate of false positives is achievable. In a population with a very low prevalence of disease, the U.S. military program for screening civilian applicants reported a false positive rate of 0.000007 (one in 135,187 persons tested).[37]

Some hospitals will not perform the test for HIV if the patient has not given informed consent. If the patient refuses consent, the probability of infection might be higher. It might seem prudent to assume that the source patient is seropositive under these circumstances. This assumption forces the health-care worker to endure mental anguish and possibly to elect toxic treatment which might not be indicated if the test were known to be negative. If one assumes that the refusal of consent means that the patient is in a group with a 50 percent prevalence of disease and an annual incidence of 10 percent, then a negative test result lowers the probability of infection from greater than 0.50 to about 0.02, i.e., by a factor of 25.

In refusing to allow tests without informed consent, the hospital is balancing several risks. One concern is liability for possible breaches of confidentiality. Alternately, the hospital might be held liable for harm experienced by injured health-care workers who must make decisions without all the pertinent information. Possible harms include adverse reactions to zidovudine, loss of consortium, or emotional distress. If the health-care worker infects another person, he or she might allege that this would not have occurred had the worker been informed of a definite exposure to HIV.

It is also possible that the courts will at some point decide that "universal precautions" are inadequate for patients or specimens known to be high risk. Clearly, universal precautions are desirable in that they decrease risk from exposure to patients whose infections are not recognized, and they may decrease the nosocomial [acquired in the hospital] infection rate due to other organisms. However, health-care workers might argue that they would have taken *additional* precautions in the face of a *known* hazard.

Conclusions

Although risk calculations must be based on a variety of assumptions that are likely to require modification as more data become available, it appears that the care of patients who are infected with HIV exposes health-care workers, especially those who perform invasive procedures, to a significant risk of infection with a disease that is highly likely to be fatal. This risk appears to be substantially greater than the risk of accidental death faced by workers in other occupations that are acknowledged to be unusually hazardous and compensated accordingly.

The risk of caring for a patient with a known HIV infection may be several orders of magnitude greater than that of caring for a randomly selected member of the population. Thus, the use of protective measures too cumbersome and expensive for routine universal precautions may be justified in patients with known infection, if they prevent less than half of all needlesticks, especially if universal precautions reduce the risk by only a relatively small fraction (less than half).

The significance of a risk is determined by many factors. The willingness of a person to accept a risk of a certain magnitude depends on his or her life situation and personal values. The ethical imperatives may not be the same for physicians as for ancillary personnel such as phlebotomists and laboratory technicians. Risk must also be viewed in the light of expected benefits. A higher risk is acceptable for lifesaving procedures than for those of marginal value.

Although the numerical risk is subject to many uncertainties and is by no means the only important consideration in making policy decisions, it is one that should not be ignored.

Notes and References

1. A revised version of this article has been published in *Southern Medical Journal*, 83 (October 1990):1121-1127.

2. Dr. Orient is in the solo practice of Internal Medicine in Tucson, Arizona. She is Chairman of the Infectious Control Committee at Carondelet St. Joseph's Hospital in Tucson. (This article does not necessarily represent the views of Carondelet Health Care Corporation.) She is also Past President

and current Executive Director of the Association of American Physicians and Surgeons. She is a widely published author.

3. D. Holthaus, "Consent Advised Before AIDS-Antibody Tests," *Hospitals*, 62 (July 20, 1988):40-41.

4. K. Henry, *et al.*, "Human Immunodeficiency Virus Antibody Testing,"*The Journal of the American Medical Association*," 259 (March 25, 1988):1819-1822.

5. Assistant Secretary For Occupational Safety and Health, *Enforcement Procedures for Occupational Exposure to Hepatitis B Virus (HBV) Human Immunodeficiency Virus (HIV), and Other Blood-Borne Infectious Agents in Health Care Facilities.* Washington, DC: US Department of Labor, (January 19, 1988). (OSHA Instruction CPL 2-2.44).

6. B. B. Dan, "Patients Without Physicians: The New Risk of AIDS," *The Journal of the American Medical Association* 258 (October 9, 1987):1949.

7. F. Rosner, "The Physician's Obligation to Heal AIDS Patients in Jewish Law," *The Journal of the American Medical Association* 260 (November 18, 1988):2837-2838.

8. Editor, AIDS Program, Hospital Infections Program, Centers for Infectious Diseases, CDC, "Update: Acquired Immunodeficiency Syndrome and Human Immunodeficiency Virus Infection Among Health Care Workers," *Morbidity and Mortality Weekly Report* 37 (April 22, 1988):229-234, 239.

9. J. Erickson, "UA [University of Arizona] Classes Help Health Workers Overcome Fear of Handling AIDS Patients," *Arizona Daily Star* (December 11, 1988):6A

10. R. Marcus, "Surveillance of Health Care Workers Exposed to Blood From Patients Infected With the Human Immunodeficiency Virus," *The New England Journal of Medicine* 319 (October 27, 1988):1118-1123.

11. G. P. Wormser, *et al.*, "Frequency of Nosocomial Transmission of HIV Infection Among Health Care Workers," *The New England Journal of Medicine* 319 (August 4, 1988):307-308.

12. J. Jagger, *et al.*, "Rates of Needlestick Injury Caused by Various Devices in a University Hospital," *The New England Journal of Medicine* 319 (August 4, 1988):284-288.

13. *Ibid.*

14. R. Wilson, *et al.*, " Risk Assessment and Comparison: An Introduction," *Science* 236 (April 17, 1987):267-280.

15. S. Hearn, B., *et al.*, "Occupational Mortality in the Oil Industry -- Louisiana," *Morbidity and Mortality Weekly Report* 29 (May 23, 1980):230-231.

16. B. L. Cohen *et al.*, "A Catalog of Risks," *Health Physics* 36 (1979):707-722.

17. Hearn, "Occupational Mortality in the Oil Industry," 230-231.

18. W. K. Sinclair, "Radiation Protection: The NCRP Guidelines and Some Considerations for the Future," *Yale Journal of Biology and Medicine* 54 (November-December, 1981):471-484.

19. *Ibid.*

20. B. Lee, "Dentists and Risk of HIV," *The New England Journal of Medicine*, 319 (July 4, 1988):113.

21. M. D. Hagen, *et al.*, "Routine Preoperative Screening for HIV: Does the Risk to the Surgeon Outweigh the Risk to the Patient?" *The Journal of the American Medical Association* 259 (March 4, 1988):1357-1361.

22. N. Padian, *et al.*, " Male-to Female Transmission of Human Immunodeficiency Virus," *The Journal of the American Medical Association* 258 (August 14, 1987):788-790.

23. M. A. Fischl, *et al.*, "Evaluation of Heterosexual Partners, Children, and Household Contacts of Adults with AIDS,"*The Journal of the American Medical Association* 257 (February 6, 1987):640-644.

24. M. A. Fischl, *et al.*, "Heterosexual Transmission of Human Immunodeficiency Virus (HIV), Presented at the Third International Conference on AIDS, Washington, DC (June 1-5, 1987).

25. E. McCray, "The Cooperative Needlestick Surveillance Group: Occupational Risk of the Acquired Immunodeficiency Syndrome Among Health Care Workers," *The New England Journal of Medicine* 314 (April 24, 1986):1127-1132.

26. Jagger, *et al.*, "Rates of Needlestick Injury," 284-288.

27. S.G. Arnold, *et al.*, "Latex Gloves Not Enough to Exclude Viruses," *Nature* 335 (September 1, 1988):19.

28. J. Huppert, *et al.*, "Latex Gloves Off in Virus Porosity Dispute," 336 *Nature* (November 24, 1988):317.

29. J.S. Carey, "Routine Preoperative Screening for HIV," *The Journal of the American Medical Association* 260 (July 8, 1988):179.

30. L. J. Guido, "Routine Preoperative Screening for HIV," *The Journal of the American Medical Association* 260 (July 8, 1988):180.

31. Anon., "Increasing Costs of Delivering Care," *On Center* (Winter 1988):11.

32. Editor, AIDS Program, 229-234, 239. (See Note 8.)

33. G. A. Hoeltge, "Groups, Videos Urge Universal Precautions," *CAP Today* (July 27, 1988).

34. Fischl, "Heterosexual Transmission."

35. S. N. Lehrman, "Study of HIV Exposure," *Medical Tribune* 30 (June 30, 1988):16.

36. Anon., "Serologic Testing for HIV Infection," *Morbidity and Mortality Weekly Report* 36 (August 21, 1987, Supplement 2S):13S-18S.

37. D. S. Burke, *et al.*, "Measurement of the False Positive Rate in a Screening Program for Human Immunodeficiency Virus Infections," *The New England Journal of Medicine* 319 (October 6, 1988):961-964.

GLOSSARY

This glossary contains terms that may not have been used in the book to help the reader understand other material on HIV/AIDS. It is comprised of medical, Biblical, and other terms.

Adultery - Sexual intercourse of a married man or woman with a person other than his/her spouse.

AIDS - **A**cquired **i**mmune **d**eficiency **s**yndrome. The late-stage complex of signs and symptoms caused by HIV.

AMA - American Medical Association.

Antibody - Proteins produced by specialized cells in the body to other chemicals (usually proteins) that are recognized to be "foreign" to the body. These proteins frequently belong to invading viruses or bacteria which are killed by these antibodies.

ARC - AIDS-**R**elated **C**omplex. Signs and symptoms of illness caused by HIV that may occur prior to the onset of AIDS. This term does not apply as frequently as it once did because more people of this category are now included under the category of AIDS.

Autologous Blood Transfusion - A blood transfusion with one's own blood, such as its being drawn and stored to be used later for elective surgery.

AZT - Azidothymidine, an earlier name for *zidovudine*.

Bisexual - One who participates in sexual activities with both sexes.

B-Cell - **B**one marrow-derived cell. One type of white blood cell that makes antibodies, the production of which is regulated by T-cells.

Casual Infection - Infection that may be transmitted in every-day activities at home, work, or in public places. Virtually a synonym for non-medical and non-sexual contact relative to AIDS.

CDC - **C**enters for **D**isease **C**ontrol, based in Atlanta, Georgia. Organized under the U.S. Department of Health and Human Services and the Public Health Service. Formerly, Communicable Disease Center.

DNA - **D**eoxyribo**n**ucleic **a**cid. The complex biochemicals that form the genetic material within the nuclei of cells.

EIA - **E**nzyme **i**mmune **a**ssay or ELISA.

ELISA - **E**nzyme **l**inked **i**mmuno**s**orbent **a**ssay. The most common screening test for antibodies to HIV.

"Expert" - Carries the same designation as "official."

Fornication - The broad general term used in Bible translations for sexual immorality. Thus, it would include adultery, homosexuality, bestiality, and any other such activities.

Heterosexual - A person who has sexual intercourse only with people (or a person) of the opposite sex.

HIV - **H**uman **i**mmunodeficiency **v**irus. The virus that causes AIDS.

HIV-1 - The official name for HIV used in the scientific litera-ture because a second retrovirus has been discovered and named HIV-2.

HIV-2 - A second HIV found mostly in West Africa. It causes illnesses similar to those of HIV-1.

Homologous Blood Transfusion - A blood transfusion using the blood of another person.

Homosexual - A male whose only sexual experiences involve other men. As a broad category, it can include lesbians and bisexuals, but has come to be used almost exclusively of men.

HTLV - A retrovirus called **h**uman **T**-cell **l**ymphotrophic **v**irus, followed by a Roman numeral to designate one of five types, e.g., HTLV-I. HTLV-III is the same retrovirus as HIV-1 or HIV.

Incidence - The frequency with which an entity *appears over a period of time* in a given population, e.g., 1/10,000 people will contract the Asian flu this winter. See "Prevalence."

"Innocent" - Refers to someone infected with AIDS who has not been sexually immoral or abused IV drugs. Of course, no one is innocent in the ultimate Biblical sense (Romans 3:23). (See Chapter 4.)

IV-Drug Abuser - A personally preferred term of the author, rather than IV-drug *user*. Anyone who uses IV drugs not prescribed by a physician is a drug abuser. The medical literature, however, refers to IV-drug "user."

Lymph Node - Localized mass of white blood cells (lymphocytes) in the body which functions to filter out bacteria, viruses, and other foreign materials and destroy them. They are present almost everywhere throughout the body, but are concentrated in the neck, armpits, and groin. They are sometimes referred to as "glands" or "kernels."

"Official" - Refers to officers or official policies of governmental *or* private agencies. The quote marks alert readers to the fact that what is official or stated by an official is not necessarily moral or a sound medical position -- a common finding with AIDS issues.

Prevalence - The frequency with which an entity is present in a population *at a given point in time*, e.g., 1/10,000 people currently have the Asian flu. See "Incidence."

Retrovirus - A virus that contains an enzyme (reverse transcriptase) that allows a conversion of its genetic material (RNA) to DNA, a reversal ("retro") of biochemical pairs. That DNA is then integrated into the DNA of the host cells.

RNA - **R**ibo**n**ucleic **a**cid. A type of genetic material found inside the nucleus of viruses and outside the nucleus of all living cells.

Seropositive - The condition in which a person's blood tests positive to the specific antibody being tested for. Relative to tests for HIV, seropositive usually means a positive test to both the ELISA and Western Blot.

STD - **S**exually **t**ransmitted **d**isease.

T-Cell - **T**hymus cell. One type of white blood cell that recognizes protein and other chemicals that are foreign to the body and makes antibodies against them. It also plays a major role in regulation of antibody production of both B-cells and T-cells. The major attack by HIV within the body is the destruction of these cells.

Traditional - In the medical sense, a longstanding and usually sound approach to medical practice, especially as a policy relates to public health. In the moral sense, a longstanding principle that usually has Biblical roots in a bygone era.

Viruses - Genetic particles that exist and multiply only within cells. They may co-exist with the cell without damage to it or they may damage and destroy the cell.

Western Blot - The blood test for HIV that is done if the ELISA is positive.

WHO - **W**orld **H**ealth **O**rganization. The medical arm of the United Nations.

Zidovudine - The first and most widely used drug against HIV.

Index of Scripture

Index of Subjects and Proper Names

Note: A comprehensive Table of Contents and Glossary is provided elsewhere in this book. This Index is supplementary to those sources of information. That is, most topics and titles listed there have not been duplicated here.

For additional copies of this book --

Special Discount Price of $8.00 a copy!!*

Buy extra copies for your pastor, your friends, your church, physicians, and health-care workers.

___ Please send me ___ copy(ies) of *What Every Christian Should Know About the AIDS Epidemic* at the Special Discount Price of $8.00 each, postage included (*for previous purchasers only). I have enclosed a check or provided MasterCard/Visa information below.

And . . . keep up with the AIDS epidemic with . . .

AIDS: Issues and Answers

A newsletter, written and edited by Ed Payne, M.D., the same author who wrote this book, and . . .

. . . the only periodical on AIDS that is explicitly Christian.

The usual price of $22.00 is discounted for book purchasers at one-half price! For only $11.00 you will receive a one-year subscription (6 issues) to *AIDS: Issues and Answers*.

___ Yes, I would like to keep track of the AIDS epidemic with *AIDS: Issues and Answers* for the next 12 months. I have enclosed a check for $11.00 or provided MasterCard/Visa information below. (Include amount for any books ordered at the Special Price above.)

Name ______________________________
Address ______________________________
City, State, ZIP ______________________________

MasterCard or Visa No. ______ ______ ______ ______
Exp. Date ____ ____

Mail to: Covenant Enterprises, P. O. Box 14488, Augusta, GA 30919